Understanding Alzheimer's: A Journey Through Causes, Symptoms, and Research

Sheena

<h1 style="text-align:center">TABLE OF CONTENTS</h1>

CHAPTER 1

Amylin Pharmacology in Alzheimer's Disease Pathogenesis and Treatment

1. INTRODUCTION

Alzheimer's disease (AD) is a form of dementia characterized by progressive memory loss and changes in cognitive and neuropsychiatric behaviors that lead to the inability to perform everyday tasks and death (1,2). There are two classifications of AD, familial and sporadic. Familial AD, representing only 5% of all cases, is inherited through mutations in presenilin (PSEN-1 and -2) and amyloid precursor protein (APP) genes, these cause the overexpression and cleavage of APP, producing excess amyloid beta ($A\beta$) protein accumulation. Sporadic AD, also known as late onset AD, is a multifactorial form of neurodegeneration where the cause is currently unknown.

The main cellular hallmarks of AD include neurodegeneration of hippocampal neurons that progressively spreads to other regions and two main pathological entities, extracellular $A\beta$ plaques and intracellular tangles made of hyper-phosphorylated tau protein (3–7). The progressive accumulation of these hallmarks is thought to lead to the progressive cognitive and neuropsychiatric decline observed in these patients (5). However, despite both tau and $A\beta$ pathology being hallmarks of AD, it is not yet fully clear whether in late onset AD, pathology is the driver of cellular dysregulation or rather a result of dyshomeostasis of more

fundamental cellular processes [11]. The latter suggests a more complex AD development, likely associated with multiple independent insults to we which we are exposed across our lifetime (8–10).

The Exposome in Late Onset AD

Although aging is the number one risk factor for development of the sporadic AD [11], AD is not a normal consequence of aging (1,12). A growing list of genes, the most prominent of which being APOE [12], are also being implicated in late onset AD. However, several environmental exposures throughout one's lifespan can independently, or in combination with aging, drive AD development. These range from traumatic brain injury [13–15], viruses [16,17] or toxins [18–21] to socioeconomical aspects such as low education levels [22], or lifestyle choices such as a sedentary lifestyle [23,24]. In fact, clinical outcomes associated with lack of exercise and poor diet, namely high blood pressure, cardiovascular disease and particularly Type II Diabetes Mellitus (T2DM), have all been linked to AD development [25–28].

The exact mechanisms that underlie the relationship between AD and T2DM remains unknown, however, both diseases share multiple commonalities as detailed previously (30). T2DM is characterized by the presence of hyperglycemia, hyperinsulinemia, and insulin resistance (31), both systemically and centrally. In fact, a consequence of systemic hyperglycemia and hyperinsulinemia is the reduction of insulin receptors within the blood brain barrier (BBB), which in turn lead to decreased insulin and glucose signaling within the brain [41–44].

Importantly, clinical reports show that diabetic patients have reduced thickness of brain regions, or atrophy, in regions affected in AD such as the hippocampus (36–38). Thus, not surprisingly, 70% of T2DM patients report cognitive impairment [32,33]. Like AD, T2DM is also associated with exacerbated reactive oxygen species (ROS) production linked with increased mitochondrial and ER stress [34–36], and activation of inflammatory cascades [37–40] within the brain. Also, of note, is the fact that T2DM and AD, albeit different amyloid proteins (amylin in T2DM and Aβ in AD) share amyloidogenesis and amyloid processing, clearing and aggregation changes as potential common pathogenic mechanisms, one in the pancreas and the other within the brain.

The assessment of metabolic hormone levels throughout normal aging and during disease states and their impact on neuronal processes may offer new biomarkers and novel directions to target therapeutics for AD. In this regard, the common pathogenic mechanism between the two pathologies and the potential relationship between the two amyloids (amylin and Aβ) in the initiation of both diseases, has been the focus of increasing research in the last decade as will be discussed throughout this review. Interestingly, data supports both a pathogenic and therapeutic role of amylin for AD pathogenesis [148,155]. This paradox highlights an incomplete understanding of mechanisms underlying this relationship. This is further exacerbated by the complex physiology of amyloids and receptor signaling system through which amyloids - like amylin -- signal (50–52). The latter is a potential source for further understanding pathophysiology of both diseases as well as a fruitful pathway for novel pharmacology development. Thus, here we summarize the current research in the area of amylin and CNS function and AD, provide up-to-date review of its receptor signaling mechanisms, and critically discuss the pharmacological paradox associated with amylin pharmacological therapy in the context of AD pathogenesis.

Although peripheral mechanisms have been suggested, satiety, energy homeostasis, and newer signaling mechanisms associated with amylin action are thought to be largely regulated via central nervous system (CNS) as will be detailed in the sections to follow.

2. Amylin and the Amylin Receptor

Amylin is 37 amino acid (aa) peptide, a part of the calcitonin family alongside calcitonin (Calc), two Calc related genes (aCGRP and bCGRP) and adrenomedullin (AM) [57]. Amylin is packaged and co-released with insulin in 1:100 (15:1, insulin: amylin molar) ratio from β-islet cells of pancreas after a meal consumption [58,59].

Amylin has an important role in energy homeostasis systemically and centrally and acts as a satiety hormone (56–59). For example, amylin serves an important glucoregulatory role by limiting insulin release from the pancreas [61,64]. Similarly, amylin inhibits local glucagon secretion in the liver, stomach, and intestine, slowing gastric emptying and, thus, nutrient absorption (56,57,61–63). In the CNS, amylin is known to sensitize leptin signaling [68,123], thus, serving an important role in energy homeostasis acutely, during meals, and longer-term, through the hypothalamic processes. These findings have been further validated in animal models in which amylin is genetically deleted [65–68]

Amylin Receptor Expression & Signaling

Amylin does not have a cognate receptor but rather signals through the native calcitonin receptor (CalcR), a class B, seven transmembrane spanning G-coupled protein receptor (GPCR). Specificity to amylin is conferred by the heterodimerization of CalcR with one of three receptor activity modifying protein (RAMPs 1-3) [71]. Thus, the amylin receptor (AMYR) is accepted to be CalcR complexed with a RAMP [71–77]. There are two isoforms of CalcR, alpha and beta (75,76), as well as three known isoforms of RAMPs, named RAMP1, -2 and -3, providing a highly complex signaling network through AMYR subtypes: AMYR1a, AMYR1b, AMYR2a, AMYR2b, AMYR3a and AMYR3b (72,76,77).

The different components that make up the AMYR have been reported in both the periphery, namely, the kidney, testes, skeletal muscle, pancreas, liver, stomach, small intestine, osteoclasts, and in dorsal root ganglia [69,70], as well as the CNS. Radioligand binding studies suggest the brain to be a region of highest level of amylin binding within the body [100]. Of note, early studies found amylin binding sites within the CNS in 1993, roughly six years before AMYR was fully characterized [76,77]. To this end, dense binding sites were originally characterized within the AP, NAc and the hypothalamus. These brain regions are linked to amylin's regulation of satiety. Additional sites of amylin of binding as well as amylin uptake, confirmed amylin-labeled radioactivity include: VTA, hypothalamus, NAc, SFO, amygdala, bed nucleus of the stria terminalis (BNST), locus coeruleus, thalamus pons, medulla, hippocampus, striatum, as well as frontal, occipital and parietal lobes

[69,77,92–96,101–104]

CalcR and all three RAMPS have been shown to co-localize in hindbrain and midbrain areas such the nucleus tractus solitarii (NTS) within the brain stem and the lateral parabrachial nucleus (LBPN), part of the pons within the midbrain [77,92–96]. Additionally, different RAMP subtypes are known to localize to different areas. For example, along with CalcR, RAMP1 has been found in the area postrema (AP), ventromedial hypothalamus (VMH) and the nucleus accumbens (NAc), caudate putamen and olfactory tubercles [95–99]. On the other hand, RAMP3 has been reported within the AP, dorsal thalamus, and subfornical region (SFO). In humans, RAMP2 is primarily expressed in the vasculature, and KO of RAMP2 is lethal [77], thus, it is less commonly studied. Together, these data suggest that RAMPs may confer regional and signaling specificity. Importantly, the study of AMYR signaling *in vivo* is further complicated by the fact that no AMYR conformation is 100% specific to amylin binding [81;82], and the fact that RAMPs are known to complex with nine different receptors, not just CalcR [85,86]. Similarly, since CalcR signals for its native ligand calcitonin, unless it is coupled to RAMPs, knockout strategies for either RAMPS or CalcR are not useful to determine AMYR signaling mechanisms [83,84]

In vitro studies, which confer most of our understanding of AMYR signaling, demonstrate that ligand binding to the AMYR activates adenyl cyclase and guanine pathways ($G\alpha_s$ and $G\alpha_q$, respectively) [75,78–80]. Either cascade is known to drive ERK phosphorylation (pERK), which has been established as a key signaling molecule in AMYR action [78,87,88]. When comparing the main AMYR subtypes, AMYR1 and AMYR3 have been reported to have similar binding affinity for amylin (101). However, some studies have shown a more diverse signaling pattern depending on the cascade activated and the cell type studied. For example, both AMYR1 and AMYR3 were shown to increase second messenger cAMP twenty-fold in Cos7 cells at similar doses. However, activation of these two receptor subtypes only led to a three to five-fold increase in intracellular Ca^{2+} and ERK phosphorylation (pERK) in Cos7 and HEK293 (98). Moreover, this study also reported that AMYR3 preferentially signaled for through Gq, driving increase of Ca^{2+} and pERK, over AMYR1 in Cos7 cells, but not HEK293 cells. Such studies highlight the complex nature of AMYR signaling even *in vitro*.

Antagonists for the members of the calcitonin family (i.e., AC413, AC66, $CGRP_{8-37}$, AC187, AC253) have been widely used to address the action of the AMYR. These antagonists are typically N-truncated isoforms of the native agonists that competitively inhibit receptor activation [89]. The most commonly used antagonist within this family, AC187, is modeled after salmon CT (sCT), where aa 35-37 are homologous to rat amylin. sCT is known to activate AMYR second to CalcR (57); additionally, sCT and amylin share a 30% aa sequence similarity (103). However, AC187 is missing the disulfide bridge found in amylin that is thought to be the biologically active portion of these peptides within the calcitonin family [90]. AC187 is found to be equally potent as an antagonist of AMYR1a and AMYR3a receptor subtypes, suggesting it cannot discriminate between the two [51, 83, 84, 91,106]. Together, these data emphasize the need for developing new AMY receptor pharmacology to deepen the mechanistic understanding of this hormone.

3. Amylin Central Nervous System Function

Hindbrain Amylin Function

Canonical amylin signaling within the CNS was first linked to the AP [78,105,106], a nucleus within the medulla oblongata, critical in the integration of neural inputs from the peripheral nervous system (PNS) that allows larger peptides, like amylin, to access the CNS. AMYR activation within the AP reduces feeding behavior via initiation of meal ending signals [107,108]. This effect is reversed by antagonist delivery [109,110]. Amylin also serves as a modulator of energy intake through the regulation of glucagon secretion, processes that are reversed by delivery of the AC187 antagonist, particularly as they pertain to glucagon secretion [111], food consumption [112], and inhibition of gastric emptying largely suggested to be mediated through vagal stimulation from AP outputs (56,58,114).

The CalcR and RAMP3 subtype most prominently co-localize within the AP to form the AMYR3 [93,114]. AMYR3 has been suggested to play a key role in amylin-mediated effects on glucose regulation and satiety signaling, shown by altered glucose sensitization and decreased inter-meal duration in the RAMP3 KO mouse (97). These findings seem to be restricted to AMYR3, as Zhang and colleagues (2011) showed that over-expression of RAMP1 does not alter feeding behaviors in mice [115]. However, as mentioned before, these results need to be weighed with caution since knockout or over-expression RAMPs may be driving changes beyond amylin signaling.

Hypothalamic Amylin Function

Amylin effects on long term energy homeostasis, as well as additional regulation of satiety mechanisms, are also mediated though AMYR signaling in the hypothalamus [116]. A transporter-mediated mechanism enables amylin crossing across the BBB [104,117] and allows for amylin effects in brain regions independently of AP mechanisms.

A key area in long-term energy regulation and body weight is the VMH. These mechanisms are primarily regulated via peripheral adiposity input signals. Similarly, amylin shows positive effects on overall energy balance and increases energy expenditure [112,118,119]. In this regard, amylin is proposed to regulate energy expenditure by increasing brown adipose tissue activity mediated through sympathetic nervous system. Mediation of sympathetic output in combination of amylin ability to reduce meal size is suggested to be key components of amylin signaling ability to reduce adiposity [118]. This effect is blocked by AMYR antagonist administration, which markedly increases body adiposity [112]. Such changes are also seen in a human RAMP1 overexpression mouse model [120]. Specifically, Coester et al. (2020) reported that RAMP1 over-expressor male mice showed increased fat mass deposits, despite displaying similar body weights than controls. Female RAMP1 KO did not show changes in fat mass, however, they showed altered plasma leptin levels compared to controls. This work suggests that AMYR1 may be important for these amylin mechanisms [121].

In fact, it has been hypothesized that functional amylin and leptin signaling are both required for these actions, suggesting a synergistic relationship. To this end, leptin sensitivity is lost during the obese and diabetic states, leading to the loss of satiation and accumulation of fat mass over time; however, amylin administration in combination with leptin in obese mice shows additive results on fat-specific weight loss over amylin or leptin therapy alone [68,106,122]. Furthermore, AMYR knockdown within the VMH results in reduced pSTAT3 signaling, whereas amylin gene knockdown mice have significantly less LepR mRNA within the VMH, as well as overall leptin insensitivity [68,123], collectively elucidating an important amylin sensitizing effect on leptin.

Another important downstream target of leptin and amylin activation within the hypothalamus is proopiomelanocortin (POMC), a precursor protein important for satiety and body weight management that counteracts the orexigenic actions of agouti related peptide/ neuropeptide Y (AgRP/NPY) neurons (117,124,125). The activation of POMC neurons within the ARC causes POMC to be converted to one of several end products, including melanocyte-stimulating hormones (MSHs), corticotrophin (ACTH), and endorphins (i.e., β-endorphin). MSH subtype alpha (αMSH) activate the melanocortin receptor subtype 4 and others (MC4R) receptors to mediate satiety [124,125]. A functional MC4R circuit has been suggested for amylin actions on satiety as MC4R$^{K314X/K314X}$ rats, a receptor loss-of-function model, showed a loss of responsiveness on feeding behaviors upon AMYR agonist therapy compared to WT mice [126]. More specifically, both LepR and AMYR have been suggested to trigger JAK/STAT3 or ERK signaling cascades within POMC neurons, respectively, to drive such effects [116,123].

Altogether this body of work highlights the amylin actions in mediating metabolic homeostasis processes. Importantly, however, amylin's actions extend beyond metabolic regulation to other processes that are relevant to aging and AD development, discussed in the section below.

4. Amylin levels and Alzheimer's Disease

The current literature on amylin signaling is conflicting regarding its role in AD pathogenesis. On one end, amylin has been hypothesized to drive AD pathogenesis. As the name suggests, amylin is an amyloid protein that aggregates *in vivo* during pathological states, thus, it is not surprising that its discovery was in aggregates in the pancreas of T2DM patients as well as diabetic cats [58,127,128]. Interestingly, amylin oligomers and plaques have been reported to be present in temporal lobes and within arteriole walls of both diabetic and non-diabetic patients with AD, as well as cognitively unimpaired patients. These aggregates have been reported to be mixed amylin- $A\beta$ plaques or amylin-only plaques [129–131]. Amylin fibrils, like $A\beta$, are toxic to β-islet cells in late stage T2DM, as well as neurons *in vitro* [132–134]. Recent work suggests that amylin may be serving as a seeding mechanism for amyloid beta in diabetic patients, thus further linking T2DMM to AD and supporting the traditional view of amyloid aggregation as a '*gain of toxic function*' mechanism in disease etiology [129,135].

The above evidence, however, is contested by studies showing negative correlations between amylin levels and disease pathogenesis. For example, Adler et al. (2014) showed that plasma amylin levels were negatively correlated with cognitive impairment [136]. Both mild cognitive impairment (MCI) and AD patients showed significantly lower levels of circulating amylin than age-matched control subjects. These findings were confirmed by others (139) (after adjusting for APOE4 allele, diabetes, stroke, kidney function and lipid profile [137]. An additional study from Zhu and colleagues (141) found that plasma amylin levels and AD risk might fall on an inverted U-shaped curve, where lower and extremely high plasma amylin concentrations were associated with increased AD risk, whereas high plasma amylin did not show this relationship. Interestingly, this study also reported that plasma amylin concentrations shared a positive correlation with temporal gray matter volume [138]. Collectively, this work suggests that, at least at the level of circulating amylin, the relationship is one that is beneficial, not pathogenetic, thus supporting a "*loss of native function*" mechanism of pathogenesis in conditions such as T2DM, as well as AD.

Amylin receptor modulation in AD models: Cognition

Several animal studies using native amylin preparations or non-aggregating forms of amylin (pramlintide acetate) [139], which shows similar pharmacokinetics and pharmacodynamics as human amylin [143], support these conclusions. Of note, pramlintide acetate therapy has shown beneficial outcomes in T2DM patients receiving insulin therapy, such as improving glycemic index, increasing weight loss in obese patients, and improving cognitive decline [140]. Of importance, and in addition, pramlintide lowers postprandial glucagon in T2DM patients [141] without inducing hypoglycemia [142]. These benefits also extend to cognition and mitigating AD-related pathogenesis.

Adler et al. (2014) found that five-week chronic infusion of pramlintide in SAMP8 mice (a model of accelerated aging) improved novel object recognition, a hippocampal formation dependent memory test. These benefits were linked to increased expression of antioxidant enzymes, and synaptic markers, including synapsin I and CDK5 [136]. This group extended this work to an APP/PS1 AD mouse model (147), where they showed that pramlintide therapy rescued hippocampal spatial memory deficits [145]. Additional studies have confirmed these findings in other mouse AD-mouse models. Both human amylin and pramlintide, in 5XFAD and Tg2576 mice, improved Y maze and MWM performance [146], an aspect that was demonstrated to be AMYR dependent [147].

As initially discussed, however, whether amylin receptor activation is beneficial or detrimental in AD is controversial. This is evidenced by data demonstrating that blocking receptor activation, thus inhibiting amylin function, is beneficial in AD pathogenesis. AC253 or cyclic AC253(cAC253) antagonists reportedly improved T-maze and MWM in 8 mos. TgCRND8 AD mice [148,149]. AC253 and cAC253 were suggested to improve memory deficits through increased synaptic markers, synapsin I and synaptophysin [148,149]. Kimura and colleagues (2016) demonstrated that high doses of (50nM) human amylin induce long-term depression (LTD) in CA1 hippocampal slices of older TgCRND8 mice, suggesting that amylin receptor antagonism would result in benefits [150]. However, it is important to note that the high dose and advanced stage of pathology in these mice could have confounded the resulting conclusions. Interestingly, the same authors reported that pramlintide application to CA1 in hippocampal slices induced long-term potentiation (LTP), important for memory formation, compared to controls, and suggested that pramlintide served an antagonist function, an aspect that is not well supported, at least *in vitro* [143].

Genetic manipulation of amylin receptor components in AD models suggest than amylin receptor activation may be detrimental in AD models. For example, a recent study from Patel et al. (2020) [151] demonstrated that depletion of amylin function via a 50% hemizygous CalcR knockdown in a TgCRND8 or 5XFAD rescued LTD and cognitive deficits in a MWM task observed in this mouse. However, it is important to note that knockdown of the CalcR is not specific to amylin action.

Amylin receptor modulation in AD models: AD pathology

Amylin and $A\beta$, both being amyloids, possess similar secondary beta-pleated sheet structures and are both degraded by insulin degrading enzyme (IDE) [134,152]; because of this, it has been suggested that $A\beta$ can bind to and signal through AMYR, specifically, AMYR3 [134,153]. $A\beta$ binding to AMYR has been proposed to be detrimental by 1) toxic intracellular signaling and 2) inhibiting amylin binding to its cognate receptor and driving accumulation of amylin extracellularly [153,154]. Furthermore, Mousa et al. (2020), proposed that amylin and pramlintide alter γ-secretase subunits, increasing their translocation to lipid rafts and increasing total $A\beta$ in TgSwDI mice [155]. However, it is important to note that while *in vitro* and *ex-vivo* work suggest benefits of AMYR blockade on amyloid-related parameters, *in vivo* studies using amylin receptor antagonists [148,149] reported the lack of changes in $A\beta$ burden nor APP processing.

Contrary to the above studies, others have reported that amylin and pramlintide administration reduce $A\beta$ plaque burden, again supporting a neuroprotective action of amylin within the CNS. Patrick et al. (2019) saw that chronic pramlintide reduced plaque burden and formic acid-soluble fraction (fibrillar $A\beta$) $A\beta_{1-40}$ and $A\beta_{1-42}$ compared to APP/PS1 saline controls [145]. The same study showed that hippocampal and cortical ADAM10 protein expression was increased in pramlintide-treated mice compared to saline controls, concluding that mediation of alpha secretase could be a potential mechanism of action of pramlintide to reduce amyloidosis [145]. In parallel, Zhu et al. (2015) saw that both human amylin and pramlintide decreased $A\beta$ plaque size and burden, and suggested decreased BACE1 activity as a mechanism, due to findings that amylin treated Tg2576 mice had reduced CTFβ cleavage products, confirmed through decreased BACE1 activity [146]. Overall alteration of APP-processing enzymes may speak to amylin modulation of APP enzyme trafficking or availability, a theory that remains to be carefully tested.

Amylin administration has also been suggested to regulate $A\beta$ clearance from the brain[146]. To this end, a single injection of either human amylin or pramlintide via IP or ICV leads to increased serum $A\beta_{1-40}$ and $A\beta_{1-42}$ 24 hours later in both mouse models, suggesting changes in $A\beta$ efflux by amylin [146]. This mechanism of Aβ clearance has been proposed to be via AMYR activation within cerebral arteries, causing vasodilation, increasing cerebral blood flow, thus increasing Aβ efflux from the brain [156,157].

Recent reports also suggest the ability of amylin to regulate tau pathology. For example, amylin has been shown to interact, via co-localization, with MAP2 and tau in hippocampal cells of individuals with AD, implicating negative protein-protein alterations that promote tau aggregation [158]. Conversely, Zhu et al. (2017) reported that amylin significantly decreased phosphorylated Ser396/Ser 404 Tau (PHF-1) and p25 in 3XFAD mice, compared to controls thus reducing pathology. Additionally, this study also found that AC253 blockade of AMYR blocked these effects [150]. However, the relationship between amylin and tau, and the impact of amylin receptor agonism or antagonism on tau pathology remains to be fully explored. Importantly, how such regulation or even which receptor subtype mediates Aβ and tau protein burden or clearance still remains unknown.

Amylin receptor modulation in AD models: Oxidative stress & inflammation

As mentioned previously, oxidative stress and inflammation commonly seen in T2DM and AD is detrimental to neuronal function, contributing to cellular damage and synaptic dysfunction [159–163]. *In vitro* data also supports a potential antioxidant function for amylin [145]. Therefore, a mechanism of action of amylin/pramlintide associated with cognitive benefits in AD could also involve such a mechanism. To this end, within the CNS, pramlintide treated SAMP8 [136] and APP/PS1 mice [145] showed a profound impact on stress-related enzymes including hemoxigenase-1 (HO1) and glutathione (GPx) and manganese superoxide dismutase (MnSOD) *in vivo* and *in vitro*.

A well-known source of oxidative stress stems from the inflammatory processes. In connection with this, Fu et al. (2017) demonstrated that AMYR activation may be involved in microglial activation. Both CalcR and RAMP3 were shown to be expressed in human fetal microglia, and their activation results in increased intracellular Ca^{2+}, an action associated with microglial activation. This effect was diminished by AMYR antagonism using cAC253 [164]. Nevertheless, like the findings for cognition and pathology, the above findings, have also been contradicted. To this end, Wang et al. (2015) demonstrated that amylin attenuated LPS induction of CD68, a proinflammatory marker, in a microglia BV2 cell line [165]. Additionally, knockdown of RAMP3, via siRNA, abolished amylin-mediated inhibition of CD68, suggesting that AMYR3 may be responsible for this relationship. *In vivo* work in the 5XFAD mouse showed lower expression of ionized calcium-binding adaptor molecule 1 (IBA-1) and diminished microglial activation. Importantly, co-administration of AC253 + amylin blocked this reduction of neuroinflammation, suggesting that AMYR activation may mediate anti-inflammatory pathways [150]. Together, while the data are conflicting, the presence of amylin AMYR in microglia suggests a direct inflammation regulatory role for this peptide that should be further explored.

5. Conclusions

The work described above supports a much more complex role for the peptide amylin than previously thought. Functions for this peptide clearly expand beyond the traditional peripheral metabolic regulatory roles to include several CNS functions, such as long-term energy balance, reward functions, and, reviewed in detail here, cognitive functions and cellular endpoints associated with AD development *(Table 1)*. The most attention-grabbing aspect of amylin research in AD is the directly conflicting reports of amylin agonism and antagonism being therapeutically beneficial in the disease. To this end, studies support both, a *'gain-of-toxic-function'* by amylin aggregation, either by providing a seed for Aβ [148,155], or driving toxicity through its receptor [150,153,164], as well as a beneficial effect of amylin or analog therapy [145–147,156,166,167]. The latter supports the hypothesis that aggregation-mediated depletion of free amylin may lead to a *"loss of native function"*, an aspect that is supported by negative correlations between free amylin and AD in human studies (142,148,168,169) (*Figure 1*).

The key to resolving some of these conflicts could lie in delving deeper into the complex amylin signaling pharmacology. This is particularly critical, given that amylin does not have its own receptor but rather signals through two subtypes of the calcitonin receptors when coupled to three potential modulating receptor proteins. Additional complexity is added to this already complicated system by the differential expression of these combinations across regions within the CNS, all of which could have slightly different affinities for the ligand. Because of this complex receptor anatomy and the lack of unique amylin receptor, the use of modern genetic tools to knock out a receptor becomes limited. Under genetic knockdown of calcitonin receptor or RAMPS one inherently disrupts both calcitonin and amylin signaling or any of the receptors that are modulated through RAMP binding, i.e., calcitonin-like receptor and adrenomedullin receptor.

Together, the above highlights a key need for "traditional" pharmacological studies, including detailed pharmacokinetics and pharmacodynamic studies of the native hormone, analogs, and existing antagonist in relation to each receptor subtype and CNS cell type. It also begets for the development of novel pharmacology development in this area, one which utilizes modern computational modeling and high throughput techniques to understand how these peptides bind to each receptor subtype and activate or inhibit it. The development of specific antagonist for each receptor subtype based would all for a much deeper understanding of amylin signaling *in vivo*.

Lastly, in relation to AD treatment, it will also become critical to determine effects of such molecules under carefully controlled $A\beta$ levels as well as carefully controlled measurements of aggregation, amyloid-beta processing, and degradation, since one can impact the levels of the other. Together, however, the study of this pharmacological paradox is an opportunity to foster deeper understanding of physiological amyloid functions and novel therapies in a disease than is unfortunately devoid of pharmacological interventions beyond those aimed at lowering amyloid-beta.

CHAPTER 2

Neuroprotective Effects of Amylin Receptor Activation, Not Antagonism, in APP/PS1 Mouse
Model of Alzheimer's Disease

1. INTRODUCTION

Alzheimer's disease (AD) is a progressive neurodegenerative disease that is clinically

characterized by cognitive decline, memory loss, mood changes, and disorientation due to

neuronal loss (1). Interestingly, 70% of patients who develop type II diabetes mellitus (T2DM)

experience cognitive decline and almost double their risk factor of developing dementia

(39,40,170–172). In addition to cognitive decline, both diseases also display CNS

hypometabolism, increased oxidative stress levels and neuroinflammation, and importantly also

share amyloid protein accumulation (24,40,173–181).Thus, understanding metabolic hormone

dysregulation in both T2DM and AD and, particularly, the crosstalk and commonalities between

metabolic peptides them can shed light into the relationship between these two diseases.

The metabolic hormone, amylin, is an amyloid protein produced by beta cells in the

pancreas that has historically been studied as gluco-regulatory peptide (182,183). Amylin

increases insulin sensitivity after meal-consumption and additionally signals for satiation and

increases energy expenditure largely controlled by hindbrain nuclei such as area postrema (AP)

(56,184,185). Amylin is also known to readily cross the blood brain barrier (BBB) (66,89) and

independently targeting and acting synergistically with other neuropeptides within the

hypothalamus like leptin and pro-opiomelanocortin (POMC) to regulate long-term energy

storage, expenditure and body weight (134).

More recently, amylin and amylin analogs like pramlintide have been linked to several

CNS processes and diseases beyond metabolic control, that include cellular events associated with cognition and AD pathogenesis (49,138,140,141,148–152,157,165,167,186–188). These

findings are validated by the fact that amylin receptor (AMYR) components, the calcitonin receptor

(Calcr) and receptor activity modifying proteins (RAMPs) have been reported across several regions in

the brain, including areas relevant to cognition and AD pathogenesis (51,78,90,93,95,109,185,189–192).

More importantly, our group as well as others have shown that plasma amylin levels correlate with

cognition and AD pathogenesis (138,139,141,148–150,157,186,187). To this end, animal models support

a role for amylin signaling in AD (138,140,148–150,157,167,168,193). Several mechanisms including

the ability of this peptide to regulate oxidative stress (OS) (148) and inflammation (187) and amyloid beta

(Aβ) processing (148,149) have been suggested as the mediators of such benefits. However, these

findings have been contradicted by other reports demonstrating that AMYR antagonism not agonism, is

beneficial in AD (49,131,151,194–196).

Aspects that may drive these conflicting reports include the complex nature of the amylin

receptor (50,197,198) and the differential expression of AMYR receptor types within brain regions

(91,185,199–202) and pharmacology in cell types (98,203). Additionally, to date, it is still unclear how

amylin therapy may be driving benefits (i.e., via direct CNS receptor binding or through the regulation of

metabolic tone). Therefore, to begin to more directly address this latter aspect and attempt to clarify the

seemingly clear paradox in results regarding amylin effects in AD pathogenesis we sought to determine

whether peripheral administration of PRAM, known to be beneficial in the APP/PS1 mouse (148), would

result in similar effects on cognition and AD pathology under central pharmacological antagonism of the

AMYR receptor.

2. Methods

2.1 Animals

APP/PS1 double knock-in transgenic mice (B6.Cg-Tg (APPswe,PSEN1dE985Dbo/J, Jackson

Laboratories) of both sexes were bred and housed in accordance with the Kent State University

Institutional Animal Care and Use Committee (IACUC). Mice were housed 2-4 mice per cage under a 12-

hour light-dark cycle. Weight (grams) was measured weekly to monitor health and effects of our treatments. Study treatments began at 5.5 months of age, prior to plaque deposition and cognitive deficits in this model, and ended at 7.5 months of age. A wild-type littermate control group of a similar age was used to determine magnitude of effect of our pharmacological treatments in APP/PS1 mice.

2.2 Treatments

All treatments and surgeries are described in APP/PS1 (Tg) were randomly assigned to four treatment groups: 1) a control group (Tg-Sal, aCSF), a group in which the amylin receptor antagonist AC187 was centrally delivered (Tg-Sal, AC187), a group that received PRAM subcutaneously as previously described (28) (Tg-PRAM, aCSF) and lastly, a group that received AC187 centrally and PRAM delivered peripherally (Tg-PRAM, AC187). PRAM was delivered using a subcutaneous osmotic pump (Alzet, model 1004) delivering a concentration of 2.27mg/ml pramlintide acetate (AnaSpec) dissolved in saline at a rate of 0.11ul/hr. This resulted in a daily dose of 6ug/day. AC187 (Abcam) was dissolved in artificial CSF (aCSF) at a concentration of 2.63mg/ml and also delivered at a rate of 0.11ul/hr. This resulted in a daily dose of 6.94ug/day. These doses were chosen based on previous data demonstrating effectiveness within the CNS (138,148,149,151,155). Control group received aCSF and Saline at the same rate and volume as the drugs being delivered. Experimental timeline is represented in

Figure 2.

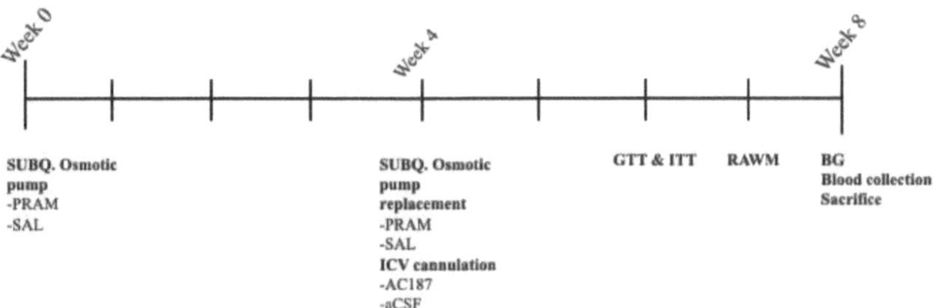

Figure 2: Experimental Timeline

Experimental timeline over 8 weeks. Week 0 is start of treatment with 28-day Alzet subcutaneous osmotic pump placement with either saline or pramlintide acetate. At week 4 original subcutaneous osmotic pump was removed and replaced with a second 28-day pump. Mice were additionally fitted with an ICV cannula into the right lateral ventricle attached to catheter tubing that was connected to a second subcutaneous osmotic that delivered aCSF or AC187. During week 6 glucose tolerance testing (GTT) and insulin tolerance testing (ITT) were performed three days apart. Week 7 radial arm water maze was performed. Week 8, fasted blood glucose levels and cardiac blood was collected at the time of sacrifice and brain tissue collection.

2.3 Surgeries

All mice in the study underwent general anesthesia (4% isoflurane) and placement of a 28-day release osmotic Alzet pump under the skin. Subcutaneous pumps were replaced once during the duration of the study at day 26 to prevent gaps in treatment as described in (28). During pump replacement, all animals were also fitted with an intraventricular (ICV) cannula and pump system (Brain Infusion Kit 3, Alzet). Briefly, animals were placed in a standard stereotaxic apparatus and the cannula was placed into the right lateral ventricle, using coordinates: λ ≤0.05mm, AP -0.05mm, ML -0.11mm and DV -0.25mm relative to bregma. The cannula was then secured with dental cement (A-M Systems) and Vetbond (Alzet). All mice were monitored daily post-operation for the remainder of the study. Correct cannula placement and functionality was tested immediately prior to sacrifice by injecting fastgreen dye solution into the line and determining coloration of the ventricle at the brain collection stage.

2.4 Behavioral testing

Spatial memory was tested using a radial arm Morris water maze (RAWM) task shown to be detect cognitive changes in the AD mouse model used in this study (204). Briefly, mice were subjected to a 120 cm pool containing six hallways with an escape platform located in the middle of one of the arms. Mice performed fifteen 60 second trials per day over two days. On day 1, trials were alternated between hidden/visible platform to speed up procedural learning. On day 2 all trials were carried out using a hidden platform. All mice were randomly assigned at goal arm with the platform in that location throughout the 30 trials. All mice randomly started each trial in different arms (except their goals arm). Visual landmarks were placed on walls of the room and served as spatial cues. Escape latency to platform (seconds) as well as number of errors committed were quantified as decedent variables. Errors were defined as 1) an entry into an arm that did not contain the platform or 2) staying in any one arm for more than 15 seconds. The last 3 trials (trials 13-15) of day 1 and day 2 were all hidden trials and were designated as probe trials. This allowed for a direct comparison of Day 1 to Day 2 errors. This relationship was converted into a 'learn score' (day 2 probe trial errors/day 1 probe trial errors) to simplify the analysis.

2.5 Metabolic measurements

Metabolic blood measures were carried out to determine potential effects of the drugs that could impact cognition and/or other measurements in the study. All metabolic blood measurements were collected after 4-5h of fasting on the day of sacrifice. ***Blood Glucose:*** Terminal blood glucose measurements were determined using a glucose meter (Contour Next) using blood collected from tail by snipping (1mm) onto a glucose strip. ***Serum Insulin:*** Roughly 300µl of blood was collected via cheek punch in tubes containing dipeptidyl peptidase IV inhibitors (DPPIV) 1:100 and Protease Inhibitor Cocktail (PIC) 1:100, to prevent the degradation of proteins. Blood was spun down at 2,000x g for 10 mins at 4°C within 30 mins of collection and serum was then collected and stored at 20°C. Insulin levels were detected in 5µl of serum/well (in duplicate) using an Ultrasensitive Mouse Insulin ELISA kit (Alpco) according to manufactures protocol. ***Glucose and Insulin Tolerance Testing (GTT & ITT):*** Tests were conducted in the mouse's dark cycle when mice are more metabolically active (205). GTT and ITT was performed at 7 months of age (a week before behavioral testing). ***GTT-*** Body weights and a baseline blood glucose measurement were taken prior to a standard glucose bolus (t_0). A standard dose of 50 mg of D-glucose in sterile .89% saline was delivered intraperitoneally (IP) based on the average mouse weight of 25g (206,207). Blood glucose was monitored at 15, 30-, 45-, 60-, and 90-minutes post IP injection as described above. Blood glucose was represented over time to depict the animals' ability to process a glucose incursion. Corrected area under the curve was calculated per group. ***ITT-*** Insulin (Sigma-Aldrich) was administered at a dose of 0.50U/kg IP injection and blood glucose levels were monitored at 20, 40-, 60-, and 80 minutes. A weight dependent dose of insulin was chosen rather than a standard dose based on a standard 25g mouse to minimize insulin shock (206,208,209). Mice whose blood glucose dropped below 45mg/dL were immediately injected with .250ml of 20% glucose and were excluded from further analysis. Corrected area under the curve was calculated per group.

2.6 Tissue collection

All animals were deeply anesthetized and quickly decapitated. One hemisphere was dissected and snap frozen for soluble $A\beta_{1-42}$ or real-time RT PCR measures. The other hemisphere was dissected and immediately homogenized in a 1X cell lysis buffer (Cell Signaling) containing 1:200 DTT (ThermoFisher), 1:100 PMSF (Cell Signaling), 1:50 PIC (Millipore-Sigma) and 1:200 protease inhibitor cocktail set III (Millipore-Sigma). Tissue was then spun down and supernatant was collected for Western blot protein analysis. Additional hippocampi were removed from an additional cohort of animals and processed for RNA sequencing.

2.7 Western Blotting- Western blot analysis was carried out as previously described in (210). Briefly, 8-12% tricine or TRIS glycine gels were loaded with 15-30ug of protein, transferred to PVGC membranes, and blotted using primary antibodies to detect protein changes in 1) metabolic proteins and receptors known to interact with amylin (POMC, LepR), 2) amylin receptor components (RAMPS, CalcR), 3) signaling molecules associated with AMYR activation or amylin signaling interactions (GSK3ß, Stat3, ERK) and 4) $A\beta$ processing (CTF α and ß, cleaved notch [γ- secretase], Arc) (*Table 1)*. After primary antibody incubation, all membranes were incubated with corresponding secondary antibodies diluted in 1X TBS-T for 1 hour at room temperature and developed using HRP Substrate ECL (Millipore-Sigma). Protein expression was visualized and captured using an imaging system (syngene) and image optical densities (OD) quantified using NIH Image J software. β-actin or GAPDH were used as loading controls.

Table 2: Chapter 2 Western Blot Antibodies
Primary and Secondary antibodies used in hippocampal and cortex tissue.

ANTIBODY	Source	Concentration	Company
β-actin	Mouse	1:5,000	Abcam
GAPDH	Rabbit	1:10,000	Millipore-Sigma
RAMP1	Rabbit	1:1000	Abcam
RAMP3	Rabbit	1:300	Abcam
CalcR	Rabbit	1:1,000	Thermo-Fisher
POMC	Rabbit	1:1,000	Cell Signaling
Arc	Mouse	1:1,000	Santa Cruz
LepR	Rabbit	1:2,000	Thermo-Fisher
CTFβ & -α	Rabbit	1:2,000	Thermo-Fisher
Notch 1 (mN1A)	Mouse	1:500	Millipore-Sigma
Ser9 GSK3β	Rabbit	1:1,000	Millipore-Sigma
GSK3β	Rabbit	1:2,000	Millipore-Sigma
Tyr705 Stat3	Rabbit	1:1,000	Cell Signaling
Stat3	Mouse	1:1,000	Cell Signaling
Anti-Mouse HRP	Goat	1:1,000	Bio-Rad
Anti- Rabbit HRP	Goat	1:1,000	Bio-Rad

2.8 Amyloid Beta Measurements

Soluble Amyloid Beta measurements - soluble (PBS), membrane bound (SDS) and insoluble (Formic Acid) amyloid beta oligomers were serial fractionalized as described by [75,76]. Briefly, hippocampal and temporal cortex tissue were homogenized in PBS with protease inhibitor cocktail at 200mg/ml and then spun down at 20,800 x g for 30 mins. This supernatant was collected and used to determine PBS-soluble Aβ content. The pellet was re-suspended in 2% SDS and again spun down as described above. The collected supernatant was then used to determine SDS-soluble Aβ levels. Lastly, the remaining pellet was homogenized in 70% formic acid in 25mM Tris, incubated for 3 hours at room temperature on an orbital shaker and spun down at 16,000x g for 20 mins. The collected supernatant was used to determine insoluble Aβ content.

Total $A\beta_{1-42}$ was measured in each of the three Aβ fractions by ELISA (Invitrogen). Briefly, all samples were run in duplicate per manufacturer's instructions. The PBS-soluble, SDS-soluble and FA-soluble fractions were run at 1:10, 1:200 and 1:50 ratios, respectively, in order to fit within each standard curve and read at 450mm on a microplate reader. Total $A\beta_{1-42}$ was expressed per mg total protein quantified by BCA assay (BioRad) and averaged per treatment group.

2.9 Real Time RT-PCR

RNA was extracted from whole hippocampus using the RNeasy mini kit (Qiagen, Germany) following the manufacturer's instructions. Concentrations and purity of RNA extracted was measured via Nanodrop. $1\mu g$ of cDNA was made using the High-Capacity cDNA Reverse Transcriptase Kit (ThermoFisher). Quantitative PCR was conducted using 10ng cDNA per reaction with the use of Brilliant III Ultra-Fast QPCR Mastermix (Aligent) and TaqMan primers (Life Technologies, CA): mouse RAMP1 (Mm00489796_m1), RAMP3 (Mm00840142_m1), CalcR (Mm00432282_m1), LepR (Mm00440181_m1), POMC (Mm07294099_m1), Arc (Mm00479619_g1). All levels were normalized to levels of a housekeeping gene Rn18S as control (Mm03928990_g1). Fold change (RQ) was calculated relative to APP/PS1 control group.

2.10 RNA sequencing

Hippocampi from an additional cohort of mice that included non-treated APP/PS1, wild-type littermates, and APP/PS1 mice treated with PRAM subcutaneously (n=3/sex/group) were collected and sent out for RNA sequencing to determine effects of PRAM on the transcriptome. All animals received the exact treatment regimen described above but did not have an ICV cannula fitted. 1 µg total of RNA was sent to the Case Western Reserve Genomics Core for RNA-sequencing. RNA quality was further analyzed using QuBit and only samples that yielded a RIN score of ≥ 8.5 were used to make RNA libraries and later used for sequencing. Processing of RNA-seq data sets were performed with Illumina NextSeq with 75 bp single-end reads at a sequencing depth of ~40 million reads on average per sample. FASTQ files containing raw transcripts were mapped to the mouse genome using HISAT2 (213), and gene expression counts were collected using Stringtie in transcripts per million (TPM) (214), using AIDD pipeline (215). Raw counts were analyzed with DeSeq2 (216) using a false discovery rate (FDR) correction cut-off of p value padj= 0.1, a relatively relaxed criterion to capture a broader set of genes, to compute differentially expressed genes (DEGs) within our comparison of interest (APP/PS1 vs APP/PS1+PRAM). All comparisons were carried out separated by sex to address sex differences in treatment. We further narrowed down the list of candidate DEGs by setting padj_value to a stricter 0.05 cut-off, together with a fold change (FC) cut-off of 1.5, a FC suggested to be biologically relevant [81,82].

Gene Expression Analysis- The TPMs from each mouse from the top 25 DEGS based on the cut-off p value between TG+ PRAM and TG+SAL mice were plotted for hierarchical clustering analysis using Heatmapper.com. Hierarchical clustering of samples using a heatmap represents the clustering of 18 (n=6/sex) mice used in this study (WT: n=3, AD: n=3; AD+ PRAM: n=3) based on their differential gene TPM expression (z-values) of the top 25 DEGs altered by PRAM compared to APP/PS1 controls. The color scale shows transcripts that are upregulated (yellow) or downregulated (blue) relative to the mean expression of all samples.

Functional gene analysis/topology-The interactions of the differentially expressed genes, with p value of 0.1, were experimentally validated with a combined score >0.7, selected as significant, and DEGs with a connection number <2 were eliminated (219). The Protein-Protein Interaction (PPI) network was visualized using GeneMANIA in Cytoscape (https://cytoscape.org/; version 3.6.8). Nodes with degree, closeness, and intermediation scores higher than the mean, calculated by the Cytoscape with CHAT and Centiscape plug-in, were considered hub nodes (220,221). To better identify and verify the molecular functions and biological processes of the identified proteins, we define the potential biological significance of the interactions an GO term enrichment was performed, using GO-TermFinder Metascape, a gene analysis and annotation resource and is displayed in REViGO (http://revigo.irb.hr/) for the elimination of redundant terms, only significant hits with a p-value ≤0.01 (222). For the GO analysis of the Hub genes, the WEB-based Gene SeT AnaLysis Toolkit (http://www.webgestalt.org/; 2017 revision) was used for the functional enrichment analysis, which covers seven biological contexts, including GO and the rate (223). FDR was set to <0.05 to perform the GO analysis of the DEGs (224).

2.11 Statistical Analysis- All behavioral and metabolic endpoint studies were blinded to the experimenter. Sex differences were addressed by powering the study to be able to detect differences in both males and female mice independently. However, to maximize our ability to detect differences a student's t-test was first performed to evaluate if a sex difference was present. If there were no statistical differences between males and females (regardless of treatment group), data were pooled and analyzed accordingly. Upon verification of normality, group differences were detected by parametric analysis using Welch or Brown-Forsythe One-way analysis of variance (ANOVA). These ANOVA tests were chosen because of uneven n numbers between treatment groups and/or unequal variance in some cases. Tukey or

LSD post-hoc tests were use when the data passed the homogeneity of variance assumption. If this assumption was not met, Games-Howell post-hoc analysis was used to report differences between groups.

3. RESULTS

3.1 Treatment effects on cognitive function

One of the main questions of this work was to address whether the cognitive benefits associated with peripheral delivery of amylin/PRAM in AD mouse models involved CNS AMYR activation or, rather, its effects were mediated through this peptide's ability to modulate the sensitivity of other key hormones such as insulin or leptin, known to impact cognition/AD-related parameters. Given the relatively young age of the mice at the end of the study (7.5 months), a T-test was first performed to validate cognitive differences between our AD model and WT. To this end, APP/PS1 mice performed more errors during probe trials than their wild-type counterparts (T= 2.402, p= 0.019), Error differences were calculated by a learning score (Day 2 probe/Day 1 probe errors) and confirmed a genotypic deficiency in learning the spatial memory task (**Figure 3A**).

An ANOVA revealed an overall significant difference of spatial memory between groups (F= 3.56, p= 0.03) when comparing all treatment groups. Games-Howell post-hoc analysis did not reveal significant differences between the APP/PS1 control group, and the PRAM treated group; however, a statistically significant difference was noted between the PRAM treated group and the AC187 treated group (p = 0.05), which performed similarly to the APP/PS1 control group (**Figure 3B**). Additionally, mice who received PRAM+ AC187 did not show differences in spatial memory compared to APP/PS1 control group nor PRAM or AC187 treated groups.

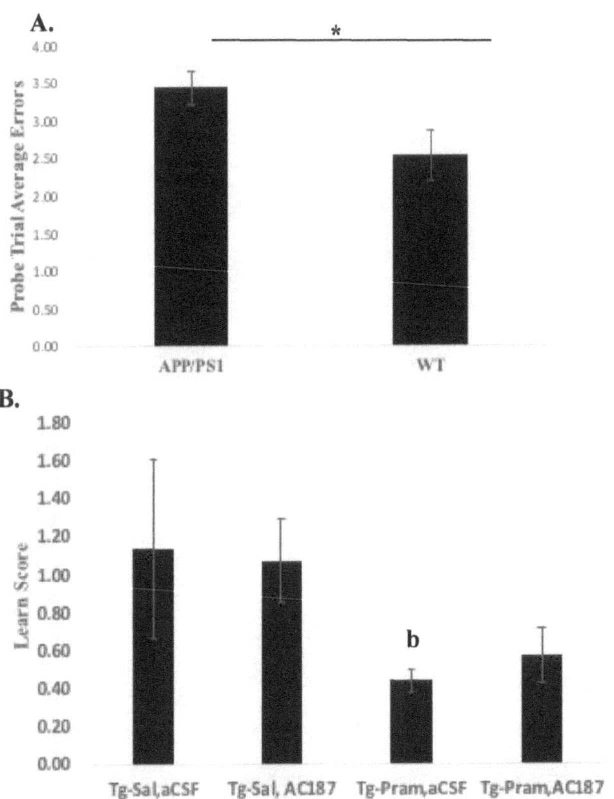

Figure 3: Radial Arm Water Maze

A. Number of probe trial errors committed between WT- Sal, aCSF and Tg- Sal, aCSF (APP/PS1) mice. * = $p<0.05$. **B**. Day 2/ Day 1 committed errors during probe trials were calculated to create a learn score for Tg-Sal, aCSF, Tg-Sal, AC187, Tg-Pram, aCSF and Tg-Pram, AC187 mice. Significance is represented as a= $p< 0.05$ compared to Tg-Sal, aCSF, b = $p< 0.05$ compared to Tg-Sal, AC187, c= $p<0.05$ compared to Tg-Sal, aCSF, d= $p< 0.05$ compared to Tg-PRAM, AC187.

3.2 Treatment effects on amyloid-beta pathology

In order to determine if CNS AMYR activation is involved in mediating amylin/PRAM reductions in $A\beta$ pathology we determined changes insoluble $A\beta_{1-42}$ species in the cortex and hippocampi of all our treatment groups. Male vs female t-test comparisons revealed sex-differences in cortical PBS (T= 2.252, p= 0.03), SDS (T= 1.807, p= 0.07) and formic acid (T= 3.163, p= 0.03) fractions, and hippocampal PBS (T= 2.258, p= 0.03), SDS (T= 3.891, p< 0.01) and formic acid (T= 2.352, p= 0.03) fractions. Therefore, ANOVAs were carried out for males and females separately.

A one-way ANOVA revealed no differences in $A\beta_{1-42}$ across treatments in male mice in either hippocampus or cortex (**Figure 3A-D**). There were also no differences in SDS-soluble treatment in females or males in hippocampus or cortex (data not shown). Interestingly, in female temporal cortex, FA-soluble $A\beta$ was significantly altered between treatment groups (Brown-Forsythe: F= 6.70, p= 0.03). Post hoc analysis shows that AC187 treated mice have significantly increased $A\beta_{1-42}$ than APP/PS1 controls (p< 0.01) as well as both groups receiving PRAM (PRAM: p= 0.02 and PRAM+ AC187: p< 0.01). There were no differences in PRAM treated (p= 0.73) or PRAM+AC187 (p= 0.98) treated mice compared to APP/PS1 controls (**Figure 3D**).

Additionally, we report that female hippocampus PBS-soluble $A\beta_{1-42}$ was significantly altered due to treatment (Welch: F= 4.6, p= 0.04). Here post-hoc analysis showed that AC187 treated mice shared a trend of increased PBS-$A\beta_{1-42}$ compared to PRAM treated mice (p< 0.075), and no differences compared to APP/PS1 controls (p= 0.99) or PRAM+AC187 treated (p= 0.60). (**Figure 3A**). PRAM (p= 0.33) treated or PRAM+AC187 (p= 0.86) showed no differences in hippocampal PBS- $A\beta_{1-42}$ compared to APP/PS1 controls.

In order to investigate these relationships further, we evaluated percent fraction of $A\beta_{1-42}$ compared to overall total $A\beta_{1-42}$ species by calculating fraction $A\beta_{1-42}$/ total $A\beta_{1-42}$. Intriguingly, in females, cortical $A\beta_{1-42}$ revealed a strong treatment effect in the percentage SDS- soluble fraction $A\beta_{1-42}$ due to treatment (F= 4.423, p= 0.02) (**Supplemental Figure 1B**). Post-hoc analysis reveals that AC187 treated mice have significantly decreased percent SDS- soluble $A\beta_{1-42}$ compared to APP/PS1 controls (p=0.04) as well as PRAM (p=0.05) and a high trend for PRAM+AC187 (p=0.06) treated mice. There were no differences in PRAM treated (p= 0.79) and PRAM+AC187 (p= 0.95) compared to APP/PS1 controls.

Furthermore, within the cortex, FA-soluble fraction/ total $A\beta_{1-42}$, one-way ANOVA showed statistically different percentage of FA $A\beta_{1-42}$ due to treatment in female mice (F= 4.729, p= 0.01) further strengthening our findings within this fraction. Post hoc analysis revealed that AC187 treated mice have significantly increased FA- soluble $A\beta_{1-42}$ compared to APP/PS1 controls (p<0.01), PRAM treated (p<0.01) and PRAM+ AC187 treated mice (p<0.01). PRAM treated nor PRAM + AC187 treated mice did not show any differences in percent FA-soluble $A\beta_{1-42}$ compared to APP/PS1 controls (PRAM p= 0.86; PRAM+AC187 p=0.90). There were also no reported differences in $A\beta_{1-42}$ percent fractions due to treatment within the hippocampus in male mice between all three fractions (**Supplemental Figure 1A-B**).

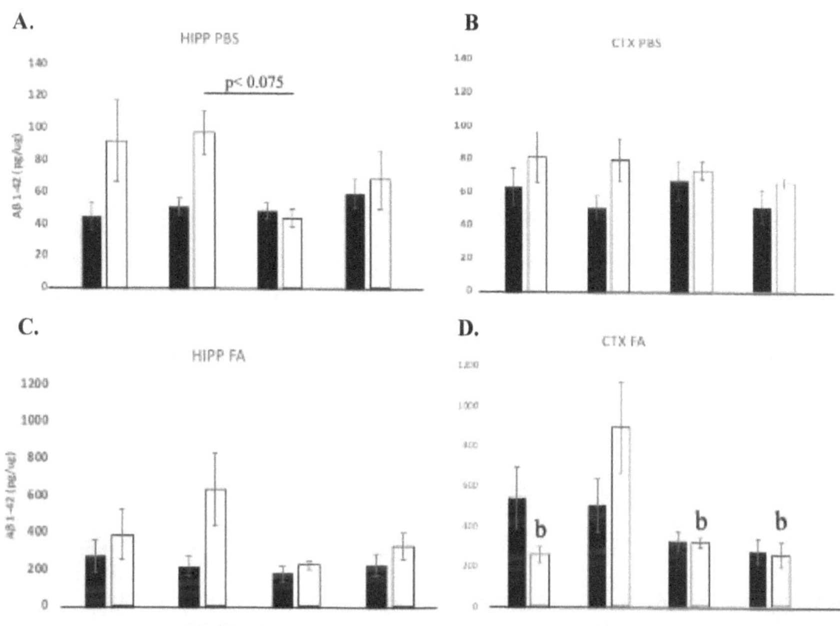

Figure 4: Soluble human A$\beta_{1\text{-}42}$ ELISAs

A. Hippocampus male and female PBS-soluble A$\beta_{1\text{-}42}$. **B.** Cortex male and female PBS soluble A$\beta_{1\text{-}42}$. **C.** Hippocampus male and female FA- soluble A$\beta_{1\text{-}42}$. **D.** Cortex male and female FA- soluble A$\beta_{1\text{-}42}$. All data represented as mean $\pm$ SEM for Tg-Sal, aCSF, Tg-Sal, AC187, Tg-Pram, aCSF and Tg-Pram, AC187 mice. Significance is represented as a= p< 0.05 compared to Tg-Sal, aCSF, b = p< 0.05 compared to Tg-Sal, AC187, c= p<0.05 compared to Tg-Sal, aCSF, d= p< 0.05 compared to Tg-PRAM, AC187.

3.3 Treatment effects on amyloid-beta processing endpoints

In order to better the understand the how AMYR activation or inhibition may alter brain $A\beta$ levels we evaluated APP cleavage enzyme activity. Specifically, α-secretase and β-secretase activity was assessed by measuring their respective cleavage products c-terminal fragments alpha and beta (CTFα and CTFβ), as well as Notch1 intracellular cleavage site to measure γ-secretase activity. Since the only differences in soluble $A\beta_{1-42}$ was found in females, we only evaluated CTFs in female mice. Surprisingly, one-way ANOVA revealed that neither hippocampal or cortex CTFβ (F= 1.856, p= 0.22) or CTFα (F= 1.986, p= 0.20) expression was significantly altered due to treatment (**Supplemental Figure 2 A-B**). Additionally, one-way ANOVA showed no differences in hippocampal cleaved Notch1 protein expression due to treatment (F= 0.537, p= 0.64) (**Supplemental 2B**).

To expand our ability to determine a mechanism for our differences in cognition and soluble $A\beta$ we also explored changes in activity related cytoskeleton-associated protein (Arc) expression since it is known to interact with APP-processing enzymes, namely PSEN1 a component of γ-secretase (225) and mediate synaptic plasticity within the dendrites of neurons (associated with improved cognition) (226–228). While there were no differences in protein expression (data not shown), mRNA transcripts were significantly altered due to treatment (F= 6.238, p= 0.01). Specifically, post-hoc analysis shows that PRAM significantly increased Arc mRNA transcripts compared to APP/PS1 controls (p< 0.01) and compared to AC187 treated mice (p=0.01). Within PRAM+AC187 treated mice, Arc mRNA transcripts did not differ from any groups (APP/PS1 controls: p= 0.11; PRAM-treated: p= 0.098; PRAM+AC187: p= 0.49). (**Figure 5B**).

3.4 Treatment effects on AMYR components & hippocampal metabolic peptide signaling

In order to determine whether the chronic treatments that we performed impacted levels of hippocampal AMYR expression and driven the significant differences observed in cognition and $A\beta$ processing, we evaluated AMYR components CalcR, RAMP1 and RAMP3 in all treatment groups. One-way ANOVA analyses revealed no differences in RAMP1, RAMP3, or CalcR protein expression in the hippocampus due to treatment (RAMP1: F= 0.753, p= 0.53; RAMP3: F= 0.830, p= 0.49; CalcR: F= 0.386, p= 0.82) (**Supplemental Fig. 3**).

Amylin is known to mediate changes in expression, transcription, and/or sensitivity of other metabolic peptides such as leptin, insulin and POMC, all linked to cognition and or AD pathogenesis. Thus, we were interested to determine how central AMYR activation or peripheral PRAM treatment altered such peptides and their downstream signaling within the hippocampus. Interestingly, our analysis showed significant treatment differences in POMC protein expression (F= 3.27, p= 0.05). Post-hoc analysis revealed no significant differences between PRAM-treated or AC187 treated mice compared to APP/PS1 controls. However, the combined PRAM+ AC187 treatment showed significantly increased POMC protein expression compared to TG+SAL controls (p= 0.04) but not to AC187 or PRAM treated mice. (**Figure 4A**).

In order to determine if changes in POMC expression were due to upstream AMYR mediated of leptin or insulin signaling we measured signal transducer and activator of transcription 3 (Stat3) activation downstream of leptin receptor (LepR), as well as glycogen synthase kinase-3 beta (GSK3β) activation downstream of insulin signaling. Overall, ANOVA revealed no changes of hippocampal long or short isoforms leptin receptor (LepRb, LepRa respectively) protein expression due to treatment. Additionally, there were no differences in phosphorylation site Y705 for STAT3 or total STAT3 protein expression associated with treatment nor on inhibitory phosphorylation site Ser9 for GSK3β (**Supplemental Figure 4A-B**).

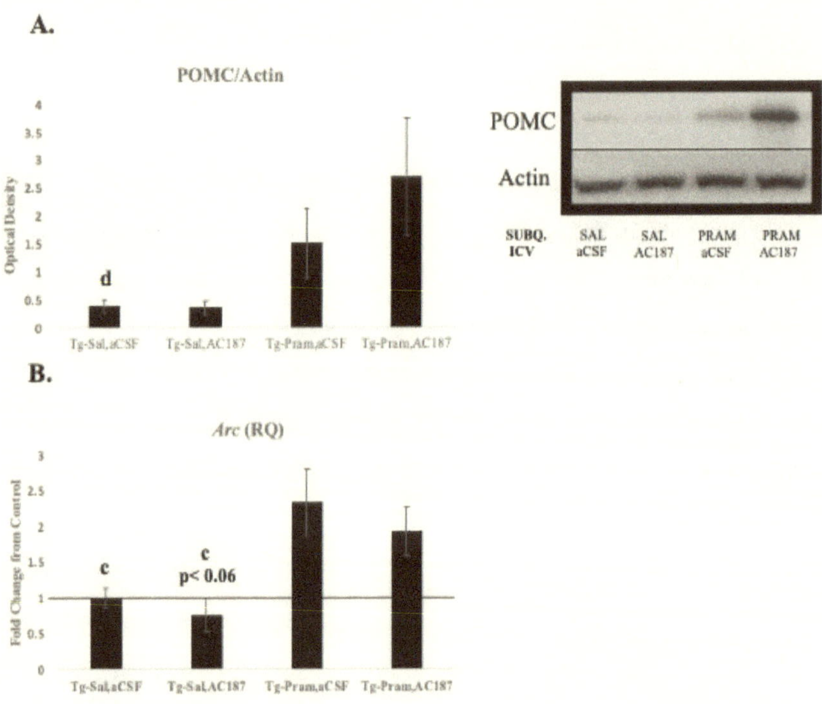

Figure 5: AMYR downstream signaling
A-B. Western blot quantification of hippocampus POMC protein expression in Tg-Sal, aCSF, Tg-Sal, AC187, Tg-Pram, aCSF and Tg-Pram, AC187 mice. Significance is represented as a= p< 0.05 compared to Tg-Sal, aCSF, b = p< 0.05 compared to Tg-Sal, AC187, c= p<0.05 compared to Tg-Sal, aCSF, d= p< 0.05 compared to Tg-PRAM, AC187. **C**. Quantative PCR quantification of hippocampus Arc mRNA transcripts. Data is represented as fold change from Tg-Sal, aCSF. Significance is represented as a= p< 0.05 compared to Tg-Sal, aCSF, b = p< 0.05 compared to Tg-Sal, AC187, c= p<0.05 compared to Tg-Sal, aCSF, d= p< 0.05 compared to Tg-PRAM, AC187.

3.6 Treatment effects on peripheral metabolic endpoints

Our treatments have been shown to have dose-dependent effects on metabolic endpoints (i.e., glucose and insulin) that can impact cognition and signaling measurements studied (229). Therefore, to be able to correlate such changes and/or use these variables as covariates in our analyses we also determined whether our treatments impacted changes in peripheral insulin and glucose levels as well as differences in insulin and glucose sensitivity. First, there was a significant difference due to sex in body weights (T= 8.91, p< 0.01), fasted serum insulin (T= 2.43, p= 0.02) and fasted blood glucose (T= 3.40, p<0.01), thus data was analyzed separately for males and females. However, ANOVAs revealed no treatment differences on body weight, fasting insulin or blood glucose levels or glucose tolerance or insulin sensitivity (**Supp. Figure 5A-E**).

3.7 Exogenous PRAM influence on hippocampal APP/PS1 transcriptome.

To expand our ability to pursue novel mechanisms, we performed RNA sequencing on hippocampal tissue of a separate cohort of APP/PS1 (PRAM and SAL-treated) and WT mice (n=3/group per sex). Differential gene expression (DEG) analysis in treated and non-treated APP/PS1 animals revealed 20 DEGs in male mice (**Table 2**), and 21 DEGS in female mice (**Table 3**) with 0 genes overlapping between the two sexes.

Within the male hierarchical heatmap, which was plotted to cross refence TPMs across WT, AD and AD+PRAM mice, of 25 genes, 12 genes in AD+ PRAM, or 48%, were "normalized" or corrected to WT male mice. Additionally, 13 genes, or 52%, were upregulated, or driven by PRAM regardless of WT or AD genotype expression (**Figure 6A**). Within the female hierarchical TPM clustering heatmap, out of 25 genes, 14 genes in AD+ PRAM, or 56%, were "normalized" to female WT mice, suggesting a rescue phenotype. Additionally, 11 genes, or 44%, were upregulated, or driven by PRAM therapy regardless of WT or AD genotype expression (**Figure 6B**).

Table 3: MALE DEGs (AD+ PRAM vs AD) padj <0.05 + FC 1.5

ENSUMBL ID	Gene	Base Mean	Log2FC	P adj
ENSMUSG00000090083	Rnf8	215.260914	-1.35	<0.01
ENSMUSG00000013622	Atraid	380.344343	-0.82	0.05
ENSMUSG00000025766	D3Ertd751e	160.394265	-1.80	0.04
ENSMUSG00000030680	Pagr1a	27.4743176	-3.01	<0.01
ENSMUSG00000029461	Fam168a	2782.3351	-0.67	<0.01
ENSMUSG00000022679	Mpv17l	741.857545	-1.34	<0.01
ENSMUSG00000032802	Srxn1	881.670474	-0.59	<0.01
ENSMUSG00000042133	Ppig	990.115893	-0.96	0.05
ENSMUSG00000046311	Zfp62	573.380175	-1.12	0.02
ENSMUSG00000029720	Gm20605	58.0811098	-3.10	<0.01
ENSMUSG00000089617	Scarna10	561.40504	-6.59	0.01
ENSMUSG00000104863		26.0546122	-4.92	0.04
ENSMUSG00000092252	Gm20499	12.1343966	-7.03	<0.01
ENSMUSG00000089865	Gm44503	19.7516965	-3.77	<0.01
ENSMUSG00000073600	Prob1	59.0158881	1.47	<0.01
ENSMUSG00000093445	Lrch4	86.4148371	2.63	<0.01
ENSMUSG00000025350	Rdh5	70.3499184	1.46	<0.01
ENSMUSG00000054752	Fsd1l	521.896711	1.42	0.01
ENSMUSG00000046836	Brox	874.924165	0.68	0.04
ENSMUSG00000025777	Gdap1	1759.47066	1.17	<0.01
ENSMUSG00000020659	Cbll1	177.38117	2.00	<0.01
ENSMUSG00000098374	Gm28043	364.23964	1.35	0.04

Table 4: FEMALE DEGs (AD+ PRAM vs AD) padj <0.05 + FC 1.5

ENSUMBL ID	Gene	Base Mean	Log2FC	P adj
ENSMUSG00000042532	Golga7b	759.622332	1.48	<0.01
ENSMUSG00000004071	Cdip1	2504.77891	0.84	<0.01
ENSMUSG00000040424	Hipk4	280.995139	0.95	<0.01
ENSMUSG00000050195	Scd4	39.0020824	4.67	0.05
ENSMUSG00000035202	Lars2	99222.6474	1.96	<0.01
ENSMUSG00000016763	Scube1	322.078798	1.30	0.04
ENSMUSG00000036339	Tmem260	312.468605	0.77	0.03
ENSMUSG00000107062	Gm43580	33.7186602	3.08	<0.01
ENSMUSG00000104953		39.205537	4.03	0.03
ENSMUSG00000106106	Rn18s	30510.5558	1.67	<0.01
ENSMUSG00000105361		74268.4612	1.92	<0.01
ENSMUSG00000038178	Slc43a2	593.473565	-1.02	0.04
ENSMUSG00000026426	Arl8a	728.6046	-0.96	<0.01
ENSMUSG00000104063	Pcdhgb7	262.399736	-1.14	0.01
ENSMUSG00000030000	Add2	4684.24464	-1.39	<0.01
ENSMUSG00000037266	Rsrp1	630.620907	-1.08	<0.01
ENSMUSG00000000794	Kcnn3	306.070181	-0.77	<0.01
ENSMUSG00000018909	Arrb1	2395.06539	-1.65	<0.01
ENSMUSG00000039850	Endov	233.765102	-1.51	<0.01
ENSMUSG00000099696	2900052N01Rik	620.173595	-0.75	<0.01
ENSMUSG00000084291	Gm6654	9.21230863	-6.62	<0.01

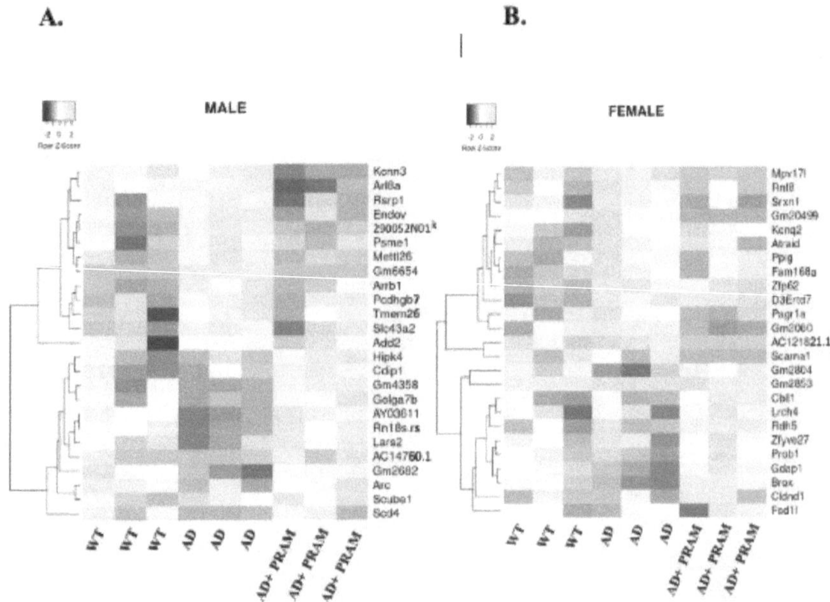

Figure 6: TPM comparisons between top 25 DEGs in APP/PS1+ PRAM treated compared to APP/PS1 controls.

A. (Male) – **B**. (Female): The top 25 genes most significantly differential expressed genes in APP/PS1+ PRAM treated mice compared to APP/PS1 were subjected to hierarchical clustering within a heatmap where TPMs from WT, APP/PS1 and APP/PS1+PRAM mice were cross referenced to determine if PRAM treatment was able to normalize the expression of any genes aberrantly affected by genotype back to the expression levels of WT mice. Color scale represents genes that were upregulated (yellow) and downregulated (blue) relative to base mean expression of all mice.

3.8 Cytoscape Interactome Analysis

In order to better understand the biological relevance of DEGs found in our analysis we sought to evaluate the protein-protein interactions of these genes through network analysis utilizing CytoScape. The interactome analysis was carried out separately for male and female mice. The parameters for the input data in both cases were the following: the results of DEGs with an adjusted p-value of 0.1 and 0.05 were taken, for each comparison in both sexes, with the predetermined confidence score of 0.4, generating a network for the males of 38 nodes and 99 edges, females 43 nodes with 63 edges. The nodes were colored in Cytoscape, based on whether they were up-regulated (yellow) or down-regulate (blue) in the DEG data. Grey nodes are the interacting neighbor genes with DEGs included in analysis by GeneMANIA in Cytoscape. Edges with high confidence scores are represented as thicker in width. For the analysis of the clusters, we use an inflation value of 2.0, to reduce the size of the clusters. The hubs of the networks were determined by Gentiscape and CHATapp in Cytoscape. In our cohort of males (**Figure 7**), the annotations indicate that there are key cluster of genes that are related to biological processes associated with the regulation of G-protein-coupled receptors (GPCRs) and with neuronal excitability. For example, the network gene is *Add2* (β-adducin), which encodes the protein Adducin 2, which plays important roles in the signaling pathways of cAMP-dependent PKA activation (Porro 2010). This supports the canonical signaling cascade associated with AMYR activation. Interestingly, the network topology in women is different from that of men. The most represented DEG cluster is associated with biological processes related to the regulation of transcription and cell proliferation, through apoptosis regulation mechanisms and DNA damage repair. The backbone of this network is the *Cbll1* gene that encodes a ubiquitin-protein E3 ligase, which fulfills essential functions in ubiquitination for endocytosis and protein degradation, as well as mediating functions in RNA processing (**Figure 8**).

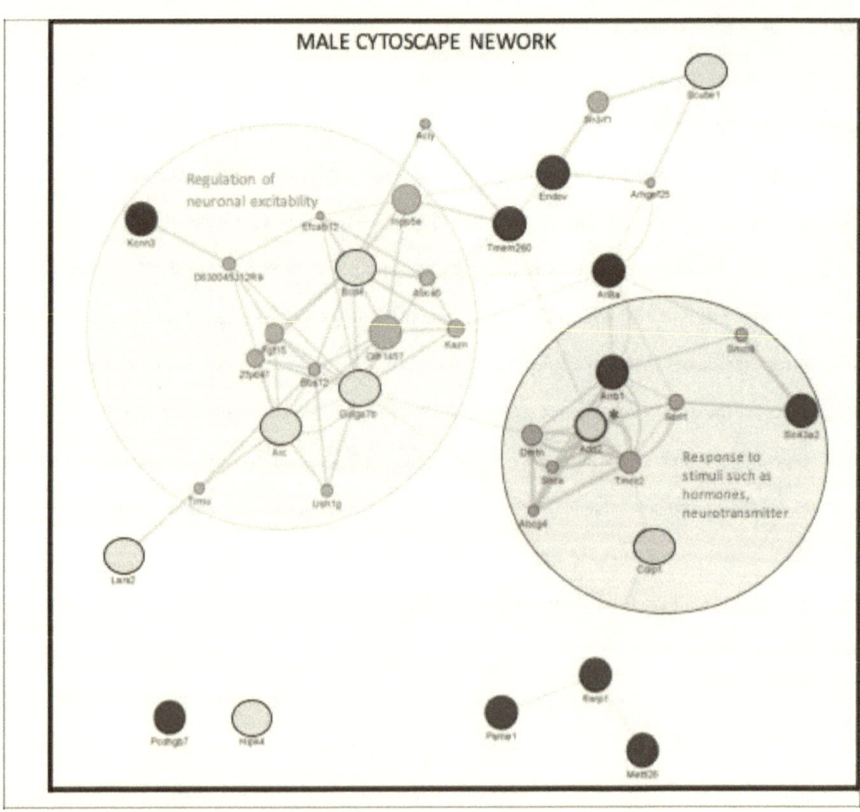

Figure 7: Male Cytoscape Topology Analysis

Male AD+PRAM DEGs with cut-off padj 0.1 + FC of > 1.5 analysis regarding functional features (Attributes, genetic interactions, psychical interactions, and shared protein domains) performed within GeneMANIA app of Cytoscape. DEGs represented as yellow (upregulated) or blue (downregulated) nodes, grey nodes represent gene interactions added by analysis. The hub gene, Add2, is denoted with a red asterisk. The main biological processes that were identified in the clusters within this network are highlighted with colored ovals, with their corresponding annotation.

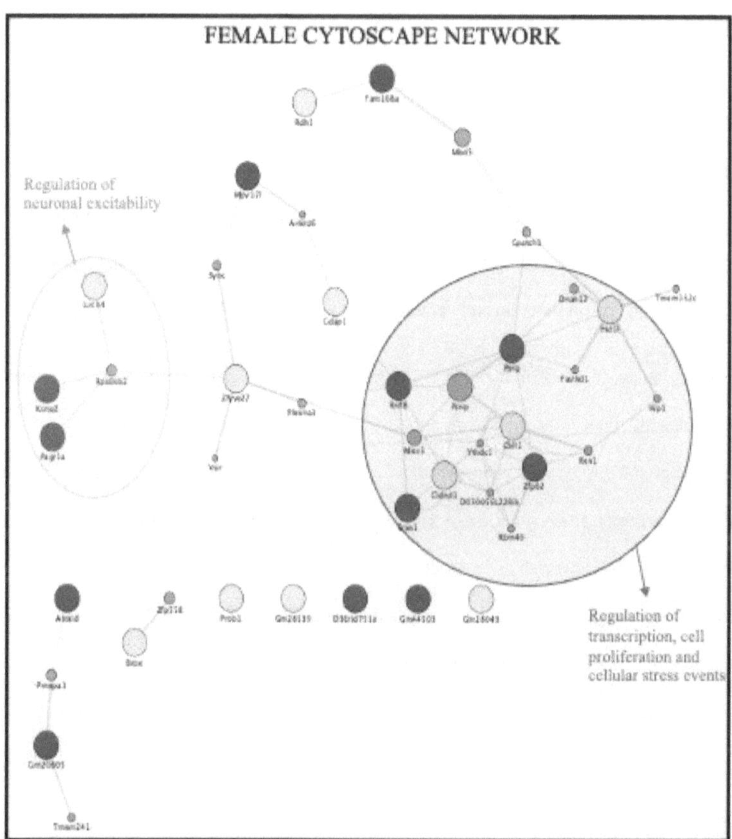

Figure 8: Female Cytoscape Topology Analysis

Female AD+PRAM DEGs with cut-off padj 0.1 + FC of > 1.5 analysis regarding functional features (Attributes, genetic interactions, psychical interactions, and shared protein domains) performed within GeneMANIA app of Cytoscape. DEGs represented as yellow (upregulated) or blue (downregulated) nodes, grey nodes represent gene interactions added by analysis. The hub gene, *Cbll1*, is denoted with a red asterisk. The main biological processes that were identified in the clusters within this network are highlighted with colored ovals, with their corresponding annotation.

4. Discussion

Here we set out to determine whether 1) the neuroprotective effects of PRAM in the APP/PS1 AD model was mediated through CNS AMYR activation or rather through its ability to regulate peripheral metabolic tone 2) potential mechanisms than could explain how PRAM is able to improve function and reduce pathology and 3) attempt to resolve the conflicting results in the literature by addressing whether central antagonism of the amylin receptor using a potent and well established AMYR inhibitor (AC187) would impact function and pathology, positively or negatively.

First, in this study, we confirm than PRAM improves spatial memory as previously published (148–150). Our data did not show a significant impact of AC187 on cognition compared to control APP/PS1. This is not unexpected given than APP/PS1 are already impaired, thus AC187 may not be able to cause further impairments. However, of note, variability in AC187 treated mice was significantly smaller than in the APP/PS1 untreated mice suggesting more consistent deficits and PRAMs benefits on cognitive function were most prominent when compared to AC187 treated mice. Thus, taken together, these data support previous published work than identified beneficial effects of PRAM on cognition but do not support the therapeutic potential for AMYR antagonism as previously reported for the antagonist AC253 (49,151,165). Route of administration, dose, animal model used, and length of treatment are all variables than can yield such differences. Also, of note, statistical power was an issue given the loss of animals during this study, however, although not significantly so, animals treated with AC187 and PRAM tended to show better function than those treated with AC187 alone. Increasing power may yield the needed resolution to further clarify these findings.

Unlike previous work, here we measured soluble $A\beta$ instead of plaque levels. This was largely since these animals were younger and thus had limited amounts of plaques to quantify. In this study, unlike previous work, our findings were restricted to female mice. This is likely because this study used younger mice and the fact that females show cognitive deficits and increased pathology earlier than their male counterparts. Using these measurements, while there was a strong trend toward significance, we were not able to detect a significant reduction by PRAM when compared to controls. However, antagonism of AMYR did exacerbate pathology. Specifically, AC187 treatment exacerbated soluble $A\beta_{1-42}$ in females within the cortex. Interestingly, within this same brain region, we saw a dramatic shift of soluble $A\beta_{1-42}$ from the SDS-soluble fragment to the FA-soluble fragment. While it is not completely understood what the SDS-soluble fraction represents in this experimental methodology, it has been suggested to represent lipid-bound, i.e., vesicle bound $A\beta$ (230–232). , These data suggest than AMYR activation is important in aspects than regulate $A\beta$ processing, clearing, or as evidenced by our fraction data, AMYR function could mediate trafficking of $A\beta$ intracellularly or even alter APP availability at the plasma membrane. These aspects will need to be addressed more directly in future studies. It is also important to consider than PRAM and AC187 may be competing for the receptor at these doses administered, at least at the level of pathology (111). More pharmacological studies will need to be performed to test this theory.

Nevertheless, to delve a little deeper into how our treatments may be affecting pathology levels we determined whether our treatments could be impacting $A\beta$ processing by C-terminal APP cleavage products (CTFs). Overall, we did not find that AMYR activation or antagonism altered the activity of APP processing enzymes. These results contradict our previous reports (148) and those of others (150) that PRAM impacted hippocampal ADAM10 and BACE1 activity. This may be partially due to the fact than animals in those studies were older and showed more robust pathology.

Changes in pathology can also occur via alterations in intracellular γ-secretase activity. To this end, Mousa et al 2020 (233) reported than PRAM altered γ-secretase activity and translocation to lipid rafts which resulted in changes in $A\beta$ pathology. Although we did not see altered γ-secretase activity via Notch1 intracellular cleavage site, PRAM may mediate the transport of APP itself or the secretases to the plasma membrane. To address this, we determined levels of the immediate early gene *Arc* which is known to mediate secretase- vesicle mediated transport of γ-secretase to the plasma membrane (225). Additionally, Arc has been suggested to mediate synaptic plasticity by way of regulating AMPAR availably within synapses (226,228). Here we report that PRAM drives Arc transcription. Importantly, AC187 did not regulate levels negatively below control levels, but PRAM administration in AC187 treated mice was able to increase levels of ARC almost to PRAM treated animal levels. This again suggests that either, PRAM uses an alternative peripheral mechanism of action, that PRAM and AC187 bind different sites or receptor subtypes, or than one outcompetes the other.

While increased Arc has been suggested to drive $A\beta$-related pathologies in AD models (234), our findings do not support this claim since PRAM reduced pathology while increasing Arc. As discussed above, Arc is an important mediator of long-term memory formation. Therefore, Arc changes in our paradigm may be associated with cognitive improvements rather than pathology. Conversely, it is plausible that increased Arc does drive $A\beta$ pathology in APP/PS1 mice, however amylin may mediate other compensatory mechanisms to combat this effect, i.e., $A\beta$ efflux or microglia degradation as suggested above.

One of the key questions than we set out to answer was whether PRAM could be mediating its beneficial effects through its ability to regulate peripheral metabolic tone or other metabolic signaling peptide than are known to interact with amylin. With regards to the first question, our findings did not reveal any metabolic differences of any of our treatments at a peripheral metabolism level. Fasting glucose or insulin nor insulin or glucose resistance were significantly different across groups. Weight was also not altered. This was somewhat surprising given the known role of PRAM in regulating insulin sensitivity. However, these findings were also not unexpected given than these animals had no metabolic impairment. Furthermore, previous studies using the same dose and route of administration have shown no differences in weight (148–150). Thus, while our ability to determine whether PRAM afforded its effects through peripheral regulation of metabolic tone, we can at least ascertain than the effects of PRAM on cognition and pathology were not related to its ability to regulate in insulin function/sensitivity as described by others (57,235,236).

Given than we found no correlations between cognitive output and $A\beta$ pathology (data not shown), we next aimed to further ascertain how amylin therapy may be rescuing spatial memory and pathologies in APP/PS1 mice. We were interested in asking if AMYR modulated other like-metabolic neuropeptides like leptin and POMC as amylin is known to do so in the hypothalamus (109,113,117,120,237,238). We hypothesized that amylin-mediated effects on cognition and AD pathology could be driven through interactions with these same neuropeptides in the hippocampus, as leptin (37,239–244) insulin (245–248) and POMC (249,250) have all been implicated independently in aspects of hippocampal synaptic plasticity and $A\beta$ and tau pathology. Surprisingly, however, we found no effects of AMYR agonism or central antagonist on Leptin receptor expression or activation of downstream phosphorylation of STAT3 at Y705, the canonical phosphorylation site for leptin action. Our results also yielded no significant differences on phosphorylation of ser9 on $GSK3\beta$, a known inhibitory site downstream of insulin receptor (IR) signaling. Although these data provide little in terms of mechanistic insight, our results fall in line with Zhu et al 2017 who reported that amylin does not alter the $GSK3\beta$ pathway, rather may mediate another tau pathway, p25-p35/CDK5 (150) or CDK5 itself (138). While we did not directly investigate this pathway, how AMYR agonism and antagonism drive CDK5 signaling and activity may be an important further direction to investigate.

Contrary to the lack of differences for leptin and insulin related mechanisms, our data showed that PRAM drives POMC expression in the hippocampus. Recently, a POMC-related/ melanocortin 4 receptor (MC4R) microcircuit has been reported in APP/PS1 mice (249,250). To this end, MC4R activation by POMC cleavage into alpha-melanocyte-stimulating hormone (α-MSH) induces LTP and decreases amyloid plaque burden, possibly through glial mechanisms. Our data suggest that amylin signaling may be the key link that initiates this POMC/MC4R microcircuit. However, while our data show that PRAM drives POMC expression in the hippocampus, it is unlikely that these signaling cascades are directly initiated within the hippocampus. Future studies will need to expand AMYR role in AD pathogenesis in examining other brain regions classically known for amylin function, i.e., area postrema and the hypothalamus. Therefore, these relationships should be explored further in future studies.

Given the sparse number of data points providing insight to specific mechanisms underlying the ability of PRAM to drive cognitive function and regulate amyloid pathology we preformed bulk RNA sequencing in a separate cohort of APP/PS1 mice treated with SAL or PRAM. Although chronic exogenous PRAM did not produce many DEGs compared to AD control mice in males or females, we are confident that with a tight stringency of padj < 0.05 coupled with a FC of at least 1.5, we were able to pick up statistically and biologically relevant genes that our PRAM treatment regimen affected.

Our data shows than several genes were "normalized" to WT by PRAM in APP/PS1 mice, interestingly these genes were different for male and female mice. This is not surprising given the very different course of disease in male and female APP/PS1 mice. However, relevant to amylin's impact on cognition and Aβ, our treatment altered the transcription of several genes relating to these functions. For example, chronic PRAM administration resulted in down regulation of *Mpv17l* (Mitochondrial Membrane Protein-Like), involved in ROS metabolism and mtDNA damage (251), as well as *Srxn1* (Sulfiredoxin 1) involved in Nrf2 (nuclear factor E2-related factor 2) (252) signaling and OS resistance (253). This suggests that chronic PRAM counteracts oxidative stress thus we may be witnessing a rescued, stress-free environment. This has been shown previously in other studies (148). These results are nicely coupled with downregulated genes *Pagr1a* (PAXIP1-associated glutamate-rich protein 1A), *Fam168a* (Family with sequence similarity 168 Member A) and *Rnf8* (Ring Finger Protein 8) which are involved in DNA damage response, (254–256) and apoptosis (257) which are processes typically driven by the presence of intracellular OS, again suggesting that PRAM may be mediating mechanisms relating to OS management. This is furthermore validated from results showing PRAM drives transcription of genes involved in oxidoreductase activity by *Rdh5* (258) and increases in mitochondrial dynamics via *Gdap1* (Ganglioside Induced Differentiation Associated Protein 1) (259). *Cldnd1* (Claudin domain-containing protein 1), another gene than was normalized by PRAM is also been reported to help combat caspase-dependent apoptosis (260). Together, these findings strengthen the rationale that PRAM works as a neuroprotectant, potentially through the regulation of OS management during disease states, specifically in females.

In males, the genes than we identified than were normalized to WT by PRAM were genes associated with membrane stability, GPCR signaling, neuronal excitability, intracellular transport and synaptic plasticity. Of note, it appears that PRAM decreases *Kcnn3* (Potassium Calcium-Activated Channel Subfamily N Member 3) transcription, a gene largely associated with neuronal excitability, suggesting the mediation of hyperexcitability in APP/PS1. Additionally, PRAM seems to drive increased expression of genes *Golga7a* (Golgin subfamily A member 7B), *Scube1* (Signal Peptide, CUB domain and EGF-like domain containing 1), *Scd4* (Stearoyl-CoA desaturase 4) all associated with membrane stability, a critical function in neuronal function (261) and an aspect reported disrupted in pathology and OS (262–264). Whether these genes are truly sexually dimorphic or simply represent a different stage of disease (less advance in males) and effects of PRAM at these stage(s) will need to be further addressed in future studies using animals of different ages.

In the functional network, representing known protein and genetic interactions based on the DEG data obtained from RNAseq, we used the GeneMania function to display and calculate the GO categories, most represented in these data, discovering for male animals (APP/PS1 treated with PRAM compared to their untreated control) two central gene clusters, one related to regulation of neuronal excitability, where we find genes that such as *Kcnn3*, a channel that is activated after hyperpolarization, thus controlling neuronal excitability, in these animals (males), it is observed that treatment with PRAM generates a down-regulated of this gene, which is interesting, in previous works it has been reported that increases in the expression of *Kcnn3* in the hippocampus of aged mice it generates memory deficits and cognitive defects (265). In the same fashion for the network of females, another gene for a potassium channel *Kcnq3* (Potassium Voltage-Gated Channel Subfamily Q Member 3), also plays an important role in the regulation of neuronal excitability, this gene is also down-regulated under AMYR stimulation with

PRAM. In APP/PS1 transgenic females, this decrease in *Kcnq2* has been shown to promote neurite outgrowth (266).

On the other hand, several genes involved in endosomal trafficking such as *Arc* (a confirmation of our RT PCR results), *Golga7b* and *Scd4* are up regulated in the male network by activation of AMYR as mentioned above, along with serving roles in membrane stability, they also to no surprise also are several related to neuronal plasticity, through different signaling pathways. For example, palmitoylated *Golga7b* is essential to prevent clathrin-mediated endocytosis of the protein plasma membrane-localized palmitoyl acyltransferase (DHHC5), which is binds PSD-95 and fulfills functions in synaptic plasticity, through the mobilization and stabilization of AMPA receptors (AMPARs) in synaptic spines (267–269). This pathway that is also regulated by *Arc*, a protein already previously described above as a master regulator in the synaptic plasticity modulating LTP, LTD and long-term memory formation via regulation of endosomal trafficking of AMPA receptors, as well as the processing APP via interaction with PSEN1, thus making *Golga7b* and *Arc* and their respective protein products key targets of interest in elucidating PRAM function of neuroprotective action. Furthermore, it has been reported that only the overexpression or pharmacological induction of *Arc* is capable of altering the transcription profile of 1900 genes, of which 100 of them have been associated with Alzheimer's pathophysiology (227,270,271).

The other key cluster represented when analyzing the DEGs in the group of males, under the activation of AMYR, is mainly related to the regulation of signaling related to receptors coupled to G proteins, such as *Arrb1* (Arrestin Beta 1) and to G-protein *Arl8a* (ADP Ribosylation Factor Like GTPase 8A) (272). The hub gene of the male network is Add2, which is another gene of vital importance in synaptic plasticity, in LTD and LTP, since this protein modulates the formation of synaptic structures such as dendritic spines, synaptic cone growths. *Add2* KO has been shown to generate learning deficits in murine models (273). These results show us two possible main nodes that are essential in memory and learning in the group of males, *Arc* and *Add2*, which are activated downstream by AMYR, which opens new opportunities to elucidate new therapies for AD, it also leaves open new questions to solve, including the mechanism involved in the activation of AMYR and memory and learning in Alzheimer's disease.

5. Conclusion

Overall, the current work generally supports previous studies in this mouse model (148) and more importantly, AMYR agonism as a beneficial pharmacological strategy in AD mouse models. In our hands, AMYR antagonism had no effect or resulted in negative effects (i.e. increases in soluble $A\beta$). Interestingly effects of AMYR antagonism shifted toward those observed after PRAM treatment when AC187 and PRAM where administered together. This suggests several possibilities than need to be explored in more detail. These include but are not limited to PRAM driving effects through AP or other unknown peripheral mechanism (i.e. microbiome), PRAM and AC187 preferentially signaling through different receptor subtypes (i.e. AMYR1 vs AMYR3) or receptor competition based on dose/time course.

Our exploration of mechanisms underlying PRAMs effects on cognition and pathology did not yield much, two exciting novel findings that will need to be pursued in future studies include, its link to POMC regulation and its ability to increase Arc levels. Both have been shown to have a direct impact on cognition and AD pathology, thus these relationships are worth pursing in more detail using combined genetic KO strategies for these proteins and pharmacology for AMYR modulation. Importantly, and in line with a beneficial role of AMYR agonism on AD pathogenesis, our RNAseq results point to mechanisms associated with oxidative stress and mitochondrial regulation and cellular and DNA repair in female mice. In the male, AMYR agonism is associated with cellular stabilization and neuronal excitatory tone. This interesting sexual dimorphism in differentially expressed genes may be confounded by the AD course acceleration in females compared to males. This aspect will need to be further addressed. However, these data, at least suggest that studies must be powered for sex differences.

Chapter 3

Amylin receptor mediation of hypothalamic hormone signaling in Alzheimer's Disease

1. Introduction

In the previous chapter, we found that central amylin signaling is important for extra-metabolic functions. Although changes in peripheral metabolic endpoints such as insulin or glucose levels or sensitivity, do not seem to drive PRAM therapy neuroprotection in AD models, it is well understood that amylin mechanisms regulating feeding behaviors and long-term energy homeostasis, that involve other metabolic hormones (i.e. insulin, leptin, POMC) are largely mediated though the hypothalamus. Thus, we aimed to determine whether AMYR regulation by the agonist PRAM and antagonist AC187 may have impacted hypothalamic signaling mechanisms that could explain our findings and those of others on cognition and amyloid pathology.

Alzheimer's disease (AD) has been referred to by some as Type III Diabetes (274). This association stems from the brains of AD patients also becoming insulin resistant much like T2DM patients (275,276). This state of hypometabolism, or decline of glucose uptake, is found in the brains of these patients' years before clinical manifestation of AD (277). To this end, patients who carried a PSEN mutation, showed a significant decrease in cerebral glucose uptake through FDG-PET imaging an average of thirteen years before cognitive decline compared to normal aged matched controls (278). The reduction in energy intake is thought to disrupt normal oxidative phosphorylation substrates (OXPHOS) cycling and cause mitochondrial stress that consequently leads to the production of reactive oxygen species (ROS) as well as decreased ATP production, the primarily source of energy for neurons. (278,279). This chain of events eventually lends to severe neuronal distress and the loss of synaptic connections [3,7–11].

It is now well established that peripheral metabolic hormones and their aberrant signaling during pathological states can have detrimental effects on the CNS as well. Importantly, T2DM and metabolic dysfunction is one of the largest risk factors for AD [12–14]. Understanding the underlying pathogenic mechanisms of metabolic dysregulation on CNS function may shed important, and much needed therapeutic avenues for AD. A key region important for brain metabolic peptide signaling modulation is the hypothalamus. Thus, understanding hypothalamic metabolic circuitry and signaling is crucial in further elucidating how hormone dysfunction may lead to neurodegeneration.

1.1 Hypothalamic peptides and their relationships in metabolic homeostasis

The hypothalamus is an important metabolic homeostatic master regulator that plays a large role in feeding behaviors and systemic energy balance. The arcuate nucleus (ARC) within the ventromedial hypothalamus (VMH) is a vital hypothalamic region for it is antinomically proximity to the third ventricle and medial eminence, a circumventricular organ enabling its ability to sense metabolic hormones and nutrients levels present within the bloodstream allowing for rapid coordination of whole-body metabolism [15,16]. More specifically, and important to this study, ARC neurons are known to sense blood amylin, leptin, insulin and glucose levels, triggering downstream signaling cascades important for healthy brain signaling. Understanding how these different metabolic neuropeptides interact and regulate one another within the hypothalamus during health and disease states is critical to understand how metabolic signals impact brain health and, for example, age-related declines. Importantly, and of key significance for this dissertation, addressing such relationships is also important to identify possible new targets for AD therapy, since most of these neuropeptides, particularly insulin (289–292), leptin (241,244,293), more recently also POMC (249,250), and the focus of this dissertation, amylin (131,138,140,148,157,187,193) have all been linked to AD pathogenesis independently of their metabolic roles. Below we describe such canonical roles as well as some of the interactions between them that could shed light into their extra-metabolic roles.

Although the interaction between all these players is significant and complex, here we focus on the relationship of these peptides to POMC regulation because this is the peptide that we have observed to be most impacted by our treatment approach in Chapter 2 in the hippocampus, and also as shown later in this chapter in the hypothalamus.

Insulin

Within the brain, insulin assists in glucose uptake, however the brain has additional glucose transporters (GLUTs), i.e., GLUT subtype 3 (GLUT3) that are not reliant on insulin or insulin receptor (IR) activation for glucose uptake, but rather for transport to the plasma membrane [17]. Outside of these roles, circulating insulin can activate IR+ neurons within the ARC nucleus which triggers stimulation of downstream regulation of neuropeptide Y/ agouti-related peptide (NPY/AgRP) and pro-opiomelanocortin (POMC) [18,19] which are orexigenic (appetite- stimulating) and anorexigenic (appetite-suppressing) peptides, respectively. Specifically, insulin stimulated IR promotes activation of insulin receptor substrate 1/ phosphoinositide 3-kinase/ protein kinase B/ forkhead box protein O1 (IRS-1/PI3K/AKT/FOXO1) pathway signaling which drives POMC transcription and inhibits AgRP [20–22] (**Figure 19A**). Like insulin, leptin is also a key mediator of metabolic homeostasis in the hypothalamus.

Leptin

Leptin is produced within white adipocytes and released in response to metabolic tone [23]. More specifically, leptin is classically known to signal through the leptin receptor (LepR), within the ARC nucleus which promotes signaling cascades responsible for producing long-term energy homeostasis and body weight management [24–27]. Moreover, leptin activation of LepR in ARC neurons is largely known to activate POMC transcription and inhibit AgRP via two pathways: 1) JAK activated phosphorylation of STAT3 causing dimerization and translocation to the nucleus where physical interactions of STAT3 binding to POMC and AgRP promoters occur [28,29], or 2) via IRS-1/PI3K/Akt/FOXO1 signaling [30,31] similarly to insulin signaling mentioned above (**Figure 19A**).

POMC & AgRP

POMC is a pro-peptide that gets cleaved into many neuropeptides including alpha- melanocortin stimulating hormone (α-MSH). It is released from POMC positive neurons in the ARC that project and act largely on second order melanocortin receptor 4 (MC4R) containing- neurons within the paraventricular (PVN), a largely anorexigenic nuclei in the hypothalamus [32]. Here MC4R stimulation plays a role in satiation behaviors as well as body weight management and energy output through regulation of brown adipose tissue [33–37]. Conversely, AgRP/NPY neurons from the ARC send projections largely innervating the lateral hypothalamus (LH), a well-known orexinergic nuclei where NPY regulates signaling cascades involved in increasing nutrient uptake [38].

Amylin's interaction with hypothalamic neuropeptides

Amylin, a peripherally made metabolic peptide described in detail in Chapter 1, regulates metabolic homeostasis through regulation of satiation, sensitizing insulin peripherally and facilitates long term energy and weight balance. Amylin mechanisms of action that control these processes are largely initiated within the AP of the hindbrain as well as the hypothalamus through independent pathways [39–43]. Hypothalamic amylin signaling through AMYR has been shown to mediate such homeostatic metabolic mechanisms of long-term energy and storage, as well as satiety through promoting POMC transcription. Exogenous amylin administration has been reported to independently increase pERK in POMC positive neurons over AgRP/NPY neurons in the ARC nucleus [39] via AMYR-dependent signaling compared to WT mice, an aspect shown to be AMYR-dependent. Moreover, this study also showed that amylin KO mice have increased AgRP fiber density within the PVN [39], potentially due to the lack of inhibition. Collectively this suggest that amylin contributes to overall metabolic status via production of POMC peptide, and the inhibition of NPY/AgRP, in postprandial states.

Apart from working independently, amylin is also known to be intimately involved leptin regulation of POMC and AgRP production, as metabolic homeostasis is constantly kept in check and balance dependent on metabolic status. As previously mentioned in Chapters 1 and 2, systemic amylin KO mice have reduced LepR mRNA as well as reduced downstream pSTAT3 signaling, a sign of reduced leptin sensitivity [44]. Furthermore, in leptin resistant obese mice, amylin treatment restored leptin- induced STAT3 phosphorylation in the VMN [28]. Collectively, these studies suggest that amylin and leptin are both needed systemically for full functionality of both peptides.

Conversely, how amylin mediates insulin and IR-activated downstream signaling in the hypothalamus or in the CNS in general is remains largely unknown. Notably, how amylin works independently [45] as well as synergistically with other neuropeptides within the hypothalamus is critical to understanding native and pathological brain function. Research suggests that amylin, leptin, and insulin are needed systemically together for full mediation of inhibiting feeding behaviors and energy balance, namely the POMC subpopulations within the ARC (316). Importantly, when any of these neuropeptides become altered under metabolic stressful conditions, energy production and overall cell survival are negatively impacted.

1.2 Metabolic dysregulation- impact on AD pathology and cognition

Altered peripheral metabolic hormones and brain glucose uptake are becoming increasingly accepted as key hallmarks of AD [46]. In addition to cognitive impairments and protein aggregation, disrupted hypothalamic feeding behaviors are also found in AD patients [47], suggesting that these mechanisms might link metabolic dysregulation to neurodegeneration. Importantly, both insulin and leptin have been studied for non-metabolic functions and both peptides, and together with amylin, are suggested to play critical roles in neurodegeneration beyond their ability to regulate metabolic/energy homeostasis. Such roles include their ability to regulate ROS production [48], inflammation [49] and cognitive decline [50,51] all directly linked to AD pathophysiology.

To this end, insulin signaling within the brain is involved in synaptic remodeling [52,53] and protection against Aβ toxicity [54]. Insulin resistance in the brain is strongly associated with AD and cognitive impairment [2,55,56]. Decreased insulin receptor (IR) sensitivity and signaling are observed in the AD [57,58]. Importantly, intranasal insulin replacement therapies show promising effects clinically by, slowing clinical decline [59] and improving glucose uptake in the frontal cortex [60]. However, chronic human insulin administration with depot (slow release) formulation has not reported the same results [60] suggesting that the pharmacokinetics of these drugs are important in treatment effectiveness.

Leptin and LepR signaling transduction have also been suggested to be involved in the function of AD-related brain regions, i.e., the hippocampus and cortex. Specifically, in the hippocampus leptin promotes neurite outgrowth [61] and adult neurogenesis [62]. Leptin is also known to facilitate LTP [63]. During states of obesity and T2D, chronic hyperleptinemia leads to overall leptin resistance (330,331). Interestingly, this relationship is also found within the CNS of AD patients as reduced LepR expression was also discovered [46]. Interestingly, clinically, several studies have reported negative correlations between peripheral leptin levels and AD [64,65], however, at least partially, this may be associated with lower weight and fat content of AD patients (334). Pre-clinical studies show that leptin replacement therapy in animal models of AD decreases $A\beta$ production, reduces tau phosphorylation and improves learning and memory [66]. However, leptin replacement as a therapeutic strategy at a clinical level is unlikely to be successful given rapid induction of leptin resistance upon treatment.

Notably, reduced POMC peptides in cerebral spinal fluid have been reported in AD patients compared to control subjects, suggested to be due to altered hypothalamic axonal secretion [67]. Additionally, POMC as well as AgRP neurons were reduced in 3xtg-AD mice, these aspects are extensively discussed in chapter 2 [68].

Like insulin and leptin, amylin is also known to mediate processes outside of metabolism homeostasis. As discussed in Chapters 1 and 2, amylin has been linked to AD both clinically and pre-clinically. However, whether amylin signaling drives some of the benefits highlighted in previous chapters via hypothalamic mechanisms and its interaction with other important metabolic peptides is largely unknown. Understanding how amylin receptor signaling mediates other metabolic neuropeptides in the hypothalamus, especially during pathological states such as AD, may shed much needed light into additional mechanisms underlying to role of amylin as well as the role of these other peptide hormones in disease pathogenesis and protection.

Such work can also broaden our understanding of how energy homeostasis mechanisms link to AD pathogenesis. Therefore, within this dissertation chapter we aimed to, for the first time, address how AMYR activation or inhibition regulates hypothalamic metabolic peptides and their signaling within the context AD and signaling that underlies relationships between leptin, insulin and POMC.

2. Methods

2.1 Animals

APP/PS1 double knock-in transgenic mice (B6.Cg-Tg(APPswe,PSEN1dE985Dbo/J, Jackson Laboratories) of both sexes were bred and housed in accordance with the Kent State University Institutional Animal Care and Use Committee (IACUC). Mice were housed 2-4 mice per cage under a 12-hour light-dark cycle. Weight (grams) was measured weekly to monitor health and effects of our treatments. Study treatments began at 5.5 months of age and ended at 7.5 months of age.

2.2 Treatments

All treatments and surgeries are described in APP/PS1 (Tg) were randomly assigned to four treatment groups: 1) a control group (Tg-Sal, aCSF), a group in which the amylin receptor antagonist AC187 was centrally delivered (Tg-Sal, AC187), a group that received PRAM subcutaneously as previously described (28) (Tg-PRAM, aCSF) and lastly, a group that received AC187 centrally and PRAM delivered peripherally (Tg-PRAM, AC187). PRAM was delivered using a subcutaneous osmotic pump (Alzet, model 1004) delivering a concentration of 2.27mg/ml pramlintide acetate (AnaSpec) dissolved in saline at a rate of 0.11ul/hr. This resulted in a daily dose of 6ug/day. AC187 (Abcam) was dissolved in artificial CSF (aCSF) at a concentration of 2.63mg/ml and also delivered at a rate of 0.11ul/hr. This resulted in a daily dose of 6.94ug/day. Control group received aCSF and Saline at the same rate and volume as the drugs being delivered. Please reference experimental timeline is represented in **Chapter 2, Figure 1**.

2.3 Surgeries

All mice in the study underwent general anesthesia (4% isoflurane) and placement of a 28-day release osmotic Alzet pump under the skin by making a small 5 mm and gently separating the tissue underneath the skin to slide the subcutaneous pump. Subcutaneous pumps were replaced once during the duration of the study at 26 days after implantation. Briefly, the tissue around the pump was massaged to release the scar tissue around it. A second incision was then created in the same area as the original incision, the first pump was gently extruded, and the new one was placed in the same opening. During pump replacement (26 days post-start of peripheral subcutaneous delivery), all animals were also fitted with an intraventricular (ICV) cannula and pump system (Brain Infusion Kit 3, Alzet). Briefly, after the subcutaneous pump was replaced, animals were placed in a standard stereotaxic apparatus and the cannula was placed into the right lateral ventricle, using coordinates: $\lambda \leq 0.05$mm, AP -0.05mm, ML -0.11mm and DV -0.25mm relative to bregma. The cannula was then secured with dental cement (A-M Systems) and Vetbond (Alzet). All mice were monitored daily post-operation for the remainder of the study. Correct cannula placement and functionality was tested immediately prior to sacrifice by injecting fastgreen dye solution into the line and determining coloration of the ventricle at the brain collection stage.

2.4 Western Blotting

Western blot analysis was carried out using the same protocol as Chapter 1. Briefly, 8-12% tricine or TRIS glycine gels were loaded with 15-30ug of protein, transferred to PVGC membranes, and blotted using primary antibodies to detect protein changes in 1) metabolic proteins and receptors known to interact with amylin (POMC, LepR, AgRP) and 2) amylin receptor components (RAMPS, CalcR), 3) downstream signaling molecules associated with LepR or IR activation (Ser307, IRS-1, Glut3) (*Table 5*). After primary antibody incubation, all membranes were incubated with corresponding secondary antibodies diluted in 1X TBS-T for 1 hour at room temperature and developed using HRP Substrate ECL (Millipore-Sigma). Protein expression was visualized and captured using an imaging system (Syngene) and image optical densities (OD) quantified using NIH Image J software. β-actin or GAPDH were used as loading controls.

Table 5: Chapter 3 Western Blotting Antibodies

Primary and Secondary antibodies used in hypothalamic tissue.

ANTIBODY	Source	Concentration	Company
β-actin	Mouse	1:5,000	Abcam
RAMP1	Rabbit	1:1000	Abcam
RAMP3	Rabbit	1:300	Abcam
CalcR	Rabbit	1:1,000	Thermo-Fisher
POMC	Rabbit	1:1,000	Cell Signaling
AgRP	Rabbit	1:500	Santa Cruz
LepR	Rabbit	1:2,000	Thermo-Fisher
Ser307 IRS-1	Mouse	1:1,000	Millipore-Sigma
IRS-1	Rabbit	1:1,000	Cell Signaling
Glut3	Rabbit	1:1,000	Abcam
Anti-Mouse HRP	Goat	1:1,000	Bio-Rad
Anti- Rabbit HRP	Goat	1:1,000	Bio-Rad

2.5 Real Time PCR

RNA was extracted from whole hippocampus using the RNeasy mini kit (Qiagen, Germany) following the manufacturer's instructions. Concentrations and purity of RNA extracted was measured via Nanodrop. $1\mu g$ of cDNA was made using the High-Capacity cDNA Reverse Transcriptase Kit (ThermoFisher). Quantitative PCR was conducted using 10ng cDNA per reaction with the use of Brilliant III Ultra-Fast QPCR Mastermix (Aligent) and TaqMan primers (Life Technologies, CA): mouse RAMP1 (Mm00489796_m1), RAMP3 (Mm00840142_m1), CalcR (Mm00432282_m1), LepR (Mm00440181_m1), POMC (Mm07294099_m1). All levels were normalized to levels of a housekeeping gene Rn18S as control (Mm03928990_g1). Fold change (RQ) was calculated relative to APP/PS1 control group.

2.6 Statistical Analysis

All behavioral and metabolic endpoint studies were blinded to the experimenter by an outside member. Sex differences were addressed by powering the study to be able to detect differences in both males and female mice independently. However, to maximize our ability to detect differences a student's t-test was first performed to evaluate if a sex difference was present. If there were no statistical differences between males and females (regardless of treatment group), data were pooled and analyzed accordingly. Upon verification of normality, group differences were detected by parametric analysis using Welch or Brown-Forsythe ANOVA. These ANOVA tests were chosen because of uneven n numbers between treatment groups and/or unequal variance in some cases. Tukey or LSD post-hoc tests were use when the data passed the homogeneity of variance assumption. If this assumption was not met, Games-Howell post-hoc analysis was used to report differences between groups.

3. Results

3.1 Treatment effects on hypothalamic AMYR components

First, to address the potential impact of long-term treatment with PRAM or AC187 on receptor expression, we examined changes in AMYR (RAMP1, RAMP3, and CalcR) expression in the hypothalamus, the main control area for metabolic regulation within the CNS. One-way ANOVA revealed no significant effects of treatment on RAMP3 (F= 1.881, p= 0.19) or CalcR (F= 1.881, p= 0.60) protein. However, RAMP1 protein expression was significantly different across groups (F= 12.701, p<0.01). Post-hoc analysis revealed a statistically significant increase of RAMP1 protein expression compared to PRAM treated (p<0.01), PRAM+ AC187 treated (p<0.01) and a high trend compared to APP/PS1 controls (p<0.06) (**Figure 14 A-B**).

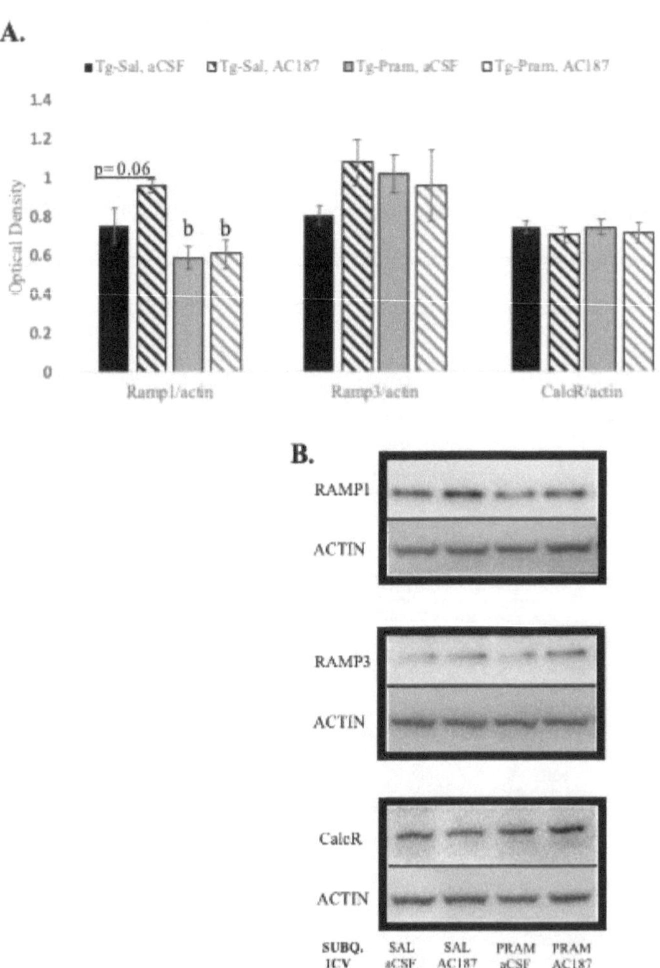

Figure 14: Hypothalamic AMYR component protein expression
A-B. Western Blotting quantification of Ramp1, Ramp3 and CalcR in Tg-Sal, aCSF, Tg-Sal, AC187, Tg-Pram, aCSF and Tg-Pram, AC187 treated mice. Data is represented as mean ±SEM. Significance is denoted as a= p< 0.05 compared to Tg-Sal, aCSF, b = p< 0.05 compared to Tg-Sal, AC187, c= p<0.05 compared to Tg-Sal, aCSF, d= p< 0.05 compared to Tg-PRAM, AC187.

Next, in order to determine if any changes in protein were due to mediation of transcription, we also evaluated RAMP1, RAMP3, and CalcR mRNA transcripts. Similar, to protein expression, Welch ANOVA showed no significant effects of treatment on RAMP3 (F= 1.141, p= 0.37) or CalcR (F= 1.942, p= 0.17) mRNA transcription (**Figure 15 B-C**). However, RAMP1 mRNA transcripts were altered across treatment groups (Welch: F= 3.443, p=0.04). Although there were no changes in RAMP1 transcripts in treatment groups compared to APP/PS1 controls (AC187: p= 0.87; PRAM: p= 0.94; PRAM+AC187: p= 0.19), post-hoc analysis reports that PRAM+ AC187 mice have significantly increased RAMP1 mRNA compared to AC187 treated mice (p = 0.04) (**Figure 15A**). Additionally, post hoc analysis revealed that RAMP1 mRNA transcripts were in PRAM treated mice showed no differences compared to AC187 (p=0.99) or PRAM+ AC187 (p=0.23) groups.

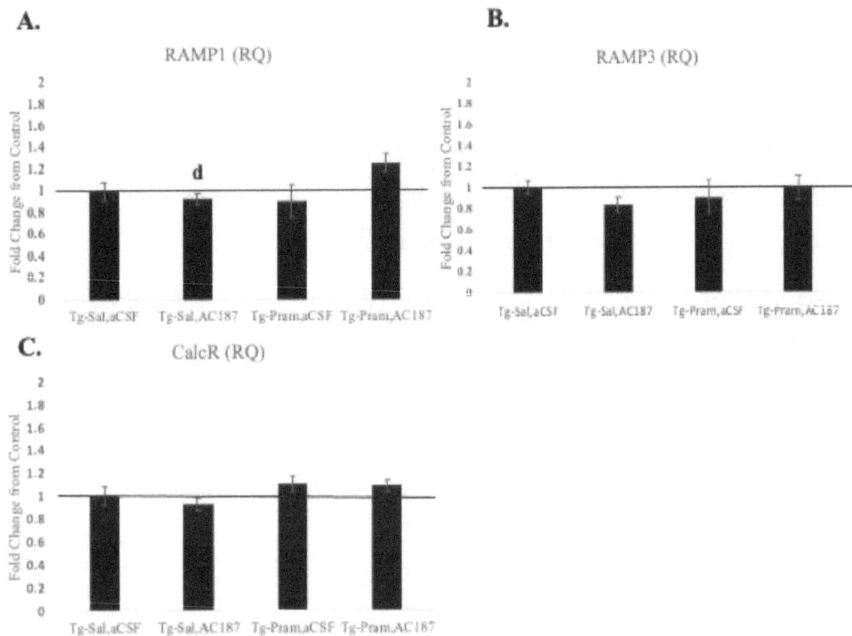

Figure 15: Hypothalamic AMYR component mRNA transcripts

A. qPCR quantification of RAMP1 mRNA transcripts in Tg-Sal, aCSF, Tg-Sal, AC187, Tg-Pram, aCSF, Tg-Pram, AC187 treated mice. **B**. qPCR quantification of RAMP3 mRNA transcripts in Tg-Sal, aCSF, Tg-Sal, AC187, Tg-Pram, aCSF, Tg-Pram, AC187 treated mice. **C**. qPCR quantification of CalcR mRNA transcripts in Tg-Sal, aCSF, Tg-Sal, AC187, Tg-Pram, aCSF, Tg-Pram, AC187 treated mice. Data is represented as fold change from Tg-Sal, aCSF controls. Significance is denoted as a= p< 0.05 compared to Tg-Sal, aCSF, b = p< 0.05 compared to Tg-Sal, AC187, c= p<0.05 compared to Tg-Sal, aCSF, d= p< 0.05 compared to Tg-PRAM, AC187.

3.2 Treatment effects on hypothalamic leptin receptor

Crucial for metabolic signaling mechanisms, we next aimed to determine whether PRAM activation or AC187 blockade of AMYR altered hypothalamic leptin signaling, a facet not previously examined in AD mice. We did so through evaluation of LepR long (LepRb) and short (LepRa) isoforms protein expression and receptor transcription. Welch One-way ANOVA did not reveal any differences of treatment on LepR protein expression (LepRb: F= 0.516, p= 0.68; LepRa: F= 0.665, p= 0.60) (**Figure 16A**).

However, LepR mRNA transcripts were significantly different across groups (Welch: F= 5.950, p<0.01). Post-hoc analysis revealed that compared to APP/PS1 controls, both AC187 (p=0.03) and PRAM+ AC187 treated (p= 0.02) groups had significantly decreased LepR mRNA transcripts. PRAM treated mice did not show differences in LepR mRNA compared to APP/PS1 controls (p= 0.25), AC187 treated (p= 0.56) or PRAM+ AC187 treated (p= 0.55) groups (**Figure 16B**).

A.

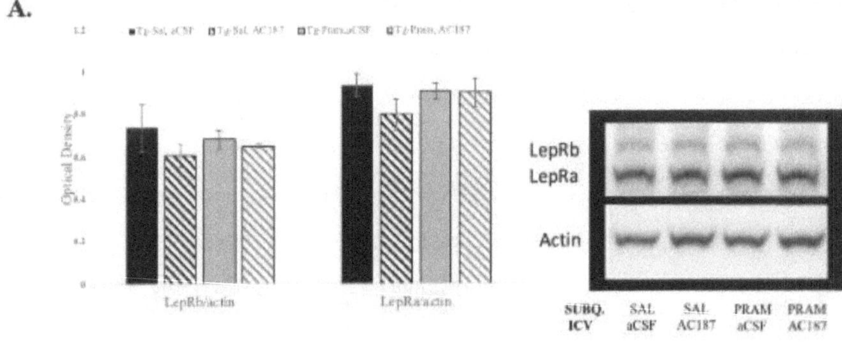

B.

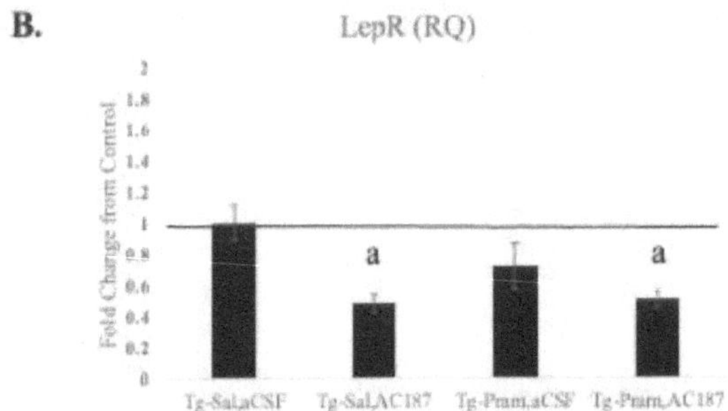

Figure 16: Hypothalamic LepR protein and mRNA transcript expression
A. Western blot quantification of LepRb and LepRa in Tg-Sal, aCSF, Tg-Sal, AC187, Tg-Pram, aCSF,

Tg-Pram, AC187 treated mice. Data is represented as mean ±SEM. **B.** qPCR quantification of LepR

mRNA transcripts in Tg-Sal, aCSF, Tg-Sal, AC187, Tg-Pram, aCSF, Tg-Pram, AC187 treated mice. Data

is represented as fold change from Tg-Sal, aCSF controls. Significance is denoted as a= p< 0.05

compared to Tg-Sal, aCSF, b = p< 0.05 compared to Tg-Sal, AC187, c= p<0.05 compared to Tg-Sal,

aCSF, d= p< 0.05 compared to Tg-PRAM, AC187.

3.3 Treatment effects on hypothalamic POMC & AgRP

Amylin and leptin both regulate POMC+ neuronal activation to increase energy expenditure and satiety within the hypothalamus. Furthermore, leptin is inhibitory towards AgRP, preventing further nutrient intake. However, these mechanisms downstream of LepR and AMYR are unknown within AD states. Thus, we were interested to determine whether chronic PRAM drives POMC and possibly modulate AgRP protein expression, or conversely, if chronic AC187 blockade would disrupt native metabolic regulation, potentially impacting neurodegenerative processes such as cognitive reserve throughout the CNS.

Interestingly we found that there was a significant sex difference in POMC protein expression where male mice overall express higher levels hypothalamus POMC than female mice ($T=17.119$, $p< 0.01$). Additionally, in males, Welch One-way ANOVA revealed POMC protein expression was significantly altered due to treatment ($F=9.921$, $p< 0.01$). Post-hoc analysis shows that AC187 treated mice have significantly increased POMC protein compared to APP/PS1 controls ($p= 0.03$) as well as TG+ PRAM ($p= 0.03$) and PRAM+ AC187 ($p= 0.02$) groups (**Figure 17 A-B**). There were no differences in male POMC protein expression in PRAM ($p= 0.93$) or PRAM+ AC187 ($p= 0.83$) groups compared to APP/PS1 controls. Additionally, Welch ANOVA revealed no differences in female POMC expression due to treatment ($F= 0.302$, $p= 0.82$).

Intriguingly however, Welch ANOVA showed no differences of treatment on AgRP hypothalamic protein expression in APP/PS1 mice ($F= 1.052$, $p= 0.44$) (**Figure 17 B-C**).

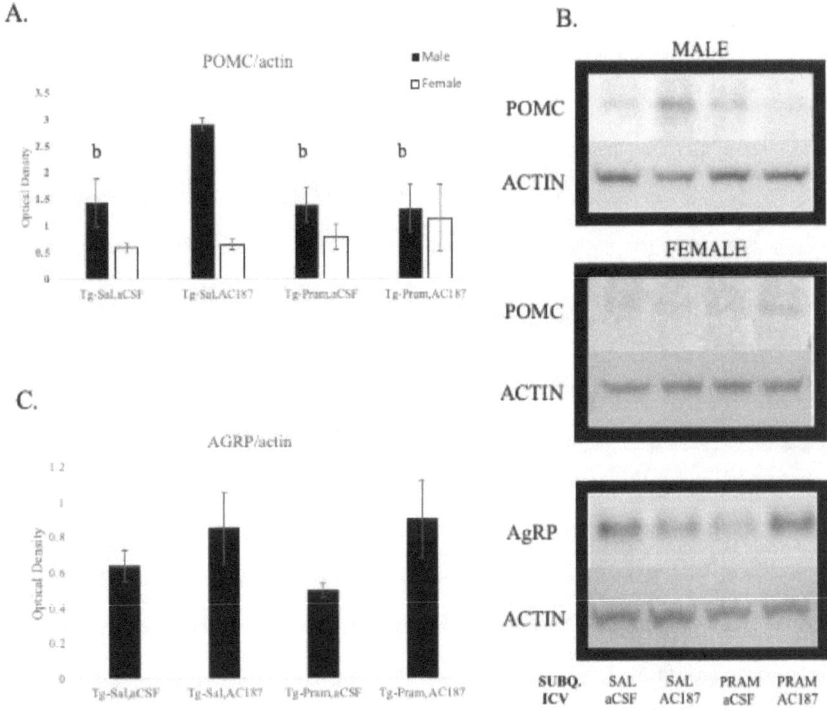

Figure 17: Hypothalamic POMC and AgRP protein expression
A- C. Western blotting quantification of POMC and AgRP protein expression in Tg-Sal, aCSF, Tg-Sal,

AC187, Tg-Pram, aCSF and Tg-Pram, AC187 treated mice. Data is represented as mean ±SEM.

Significance is denoted as a= p< 0.05 compared to Tg-Sal, aCSF, b = p< 0.05 compared to Tg-Sal,

AC187, c= p<0.05 compared to Tg-Sal, aCSF, d= p< 0.05 compared to Tg-PRAM, AC187.

3.4 Treatment effects on hypothalamic Leptin and Insulin Downstream Signaling

Amylin can mediate downstream LepR STAT3 phosphorylation which lends to POMC transcription and AgRP inhibition; however, it is unknown whether AMYR signaling is upstream of leptin and insulin regulation of POMC and AgRP transcription through IRS-1 mediated PI3K/Akt pathway activation. Furthermore, it is unknown if these specific hypothalamic pathways are altered in APP/PS1 mice. Thus, we measured total IRS-1 protein expression as well as inhibitory phosphorylation site Ser307. Overall, Welch One-way ANOVA revealed there were no changes in phosphorylation of Ser307 IRS-1 relative to total IRS-1 due to treatment (F= 0.297, p=0.83). However, Welch ANOVA showed significant differences of treatment on total IRS-1 protein (F= 6.511, p< 0.01). Post-hoc analysis shows that AC187 treated mice have significantly increased IRS-1 protein compared to PRAM (p<0.01) and PRAM+ AC187 (p<0.01) groups, as well as a high trend compared to APP/PS1 controls (p= 0.06) (**Figure 18 A-B**).

Amylin is known to increase insulin sensitivity in the periphery; thus, we were interested in investigating whether or not amylin signaling mediated glucose uptake mechanisms in the hypothalamus, as hypometabolic is a well-known metabolic dysfunction consequence during AD etiology. Thus, we also measured hypothalamic Glut3 protein expression. Welch One-way ANOVA revealed no changes due to treatment of Glut3 expression (F= 0.782, p= 0.52) (**Figure 18 A-B**).

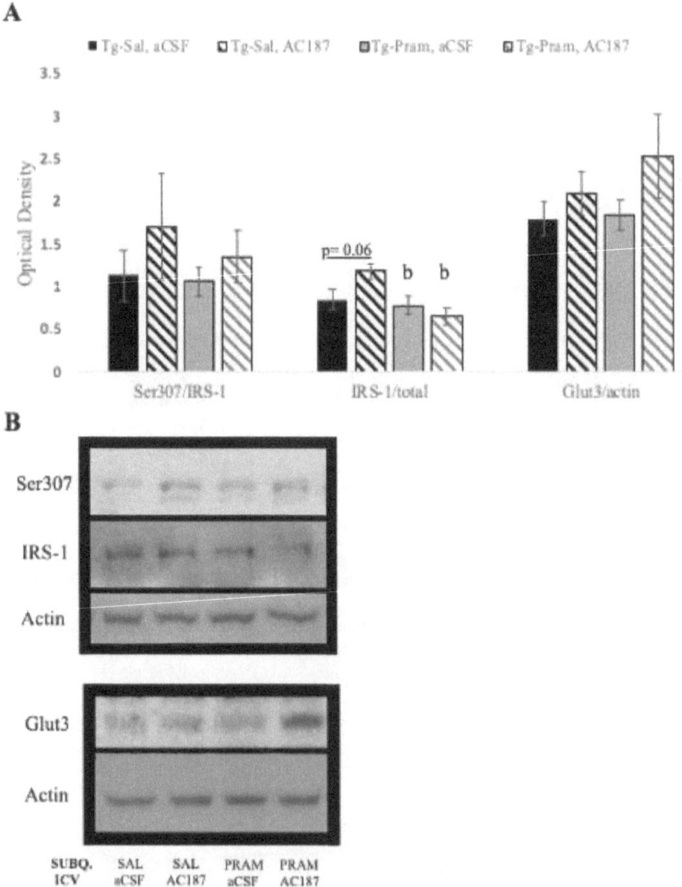

Figure 18: Hypothalamus metabolic signaling

A- B. Western blotting quantification of Ser307/IRS-1, IRS-1 and Glut3 protein expression in Tg-Sal, aCSF, Tg-Sal, AC187, Tg-Pram, aCSF and Tg-Pram, AC187 treated mice. Data is represented as mean ±SEM. Significance is denoted as a= $p < 0.05$ compared to Tg-Sal, aCSF, b = $p < 0.05$ compared to Tg-Sal, AC187, c= $p < 0.05$ compared to Tg-Sal, aCSF, d= $p < 0.05$ compared to Tg-PRAM, AC187.

4   Discussion:

To begin to address the potential mechanisms of amylin signaling than underly its ability to regulate cognition and AD pathology, here we aimed to determine whether amylin receptor activation or inhibition caused changes in hypothalamic metabolic neuropeptides, their receptors and downstream signaling associated with such peptides. More specifically, we aimed to evaluate how PRAM or the AMYR antagonist AC187 interacts with other metabolic neuropeptides leptin [39,41,69–74], IRS-1 activation and POMC/AgRP transcription because of their documented extra-metabolic functions such as cognition [2,63,75], neuronal plasticity [52,53], their extensively documented relationship with AD development and pathology [2,54,55,66,76].

Largely mimicking the lack of peripheral metabolic endpoint alterations (body weight, glucose levels, insulin levels, and GTT and ITT performance) shown in Chapter 2, PRAM treatment did not modify hypothalamic signaling in APP/PS1 mice. Although it is well known that amylin can independently increase POMC mRNA in addition to synergistically increase leptin-mediated pSTAT3 signaling regulation of POMC/AgRP regulation, we did not witness this. This was unexpected as we saw PRAM drove POMC expression in the hippocampus, thus the thought was this signaling transduction may have initiated from AMYR mediation in the hypothalamus. Moreover, we also did not see that AMYR activation altered LepR expression, although this may not be an unexpected finding since amylin has only been shown to increase leptin binding or sensitivity in states of leptin resistance and obesity. Under normal circumstances these neuropeptides are under strict equilibrium in order to balance metabolic homeostasis, thus unless disrupted by pathological states such as obesity and/or insulin resistance, treatment effects may be more difficult to detect. Future studies should determine these changes in animals than under metabolic stress.

In this study, unlike what we observed in the hippocampus (Chapter 2), we did not witness any effects of PRAM on POMC transcription or expression. However, surprisingly, we do report alterations under conditions of AMYR blockade. To this end, POMC protein expression was increased by AC187 antagonism compared to APP/PS1 controls. This effect was also observed when PRAM and AC187 were delivered together, suggesting that, unlike for all other markers surveyed in this dissertation, PRAM was not able to rescue the effects of AC187 on POMC expression. While we would not hypothesize that AMYR blockade would drive POMC expression, this finding may be explained by changes in LepR transcription than we also observed in AC187 treated animals compared to controls. Here we report similar findings as Turek et al 2010 [44], showing that loss of amylin signaling, in our case with AC187, resulted in decreased overall LepR mRNA expression. This finding is of significance because it confirms the validity of our experimental drug model.

We were further interested in determining whether alterations of POMC expression due to AC187 blockade was mediated from a commonly well-known LepR/IR activation of IRS-1/ PI3K/Akt/FOXO1 signaling pathway, an important pathway altered in T2DM and glycometabolism [77] that may also play a role in oxidative stress resistance [78]. Interestingly, AMYR blockade altered overall IRS-1 expression compared to PRAM mice, in addition to, APP/PS1 controls. These data suggest than the loss of amylin signaling, through direct AMYR signaling or reduced insulin and leptin signaling (**Figure 19B**), may drive translation of IRS-1 as a compensatory mechanism. Interestingly, translocation of FOXO1 due to Akt phosphorylation downstream of IRS-1 activation, allows for normal POMC transcription. Such a mechanism could explain why we saw increased POMC in AC187 treated mice. However, direct measurement of a stimulatory IRS-1 phosphorylation site as we all PI3K/ Akt activation and staining for FOXO1 localization would strengthen our overall findings suggesting that AMYR signaling, or a lack thereof, alters this specific signaling cascade. Furthermore, within this study, hypothalamic RAMP1 protein expression was also significantly altered in AC187 mice. Although AC187 has not been previously reported to increase AMYR expression, we offer here that this could also be compensatory for the antagonism of chronic AMYR signaling. Coester et al 2020 [80], recently suggested RAMP1 (AMYR1) to be important for amylin mediation of fat-mass utilization and long-term energy storage, mechanisms that closely tie hypothalamic amylin, leptin and POMC signaling together. Thus, preservation of AMYR availability through increased RAMP1 may be of benefit.

Altogether, the changes within hypothalamic signaling due to AC187 receptor blockade, in large do not offer any insight into PRAM mediated benefits on AD pathology within the hippocampus or cortex, however, provide a potential mechanism than can indirectly impact hippocampal function. Also, in relation to this, a limitation of this study design was the fact than ICV administration of AC187 inhibits AMYR action throughout the entire CNS, thus prevents us to address directly if any changes in hypothalamic signaling due to AC187 blockade in fact affected AD outputs measured in hippocampi or cortex from Chapter 2. Future studies warrant the direct blockade of AMYR function within the hypothalamus and then measure hippocampal and cortex measurements. This would not only possibly elucidate mechanisms of amylin neuroprotection but additionally reveal hypothalamic amylin-related circuity to higher-order brain regions, an unexplored connection.

A.　　　　　　　　　　　　　　　　　　B.

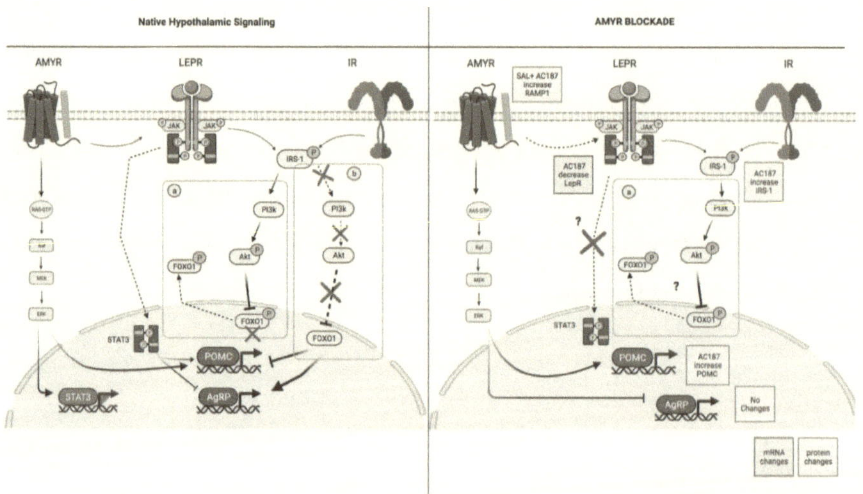

Figure 19: Hypothalamic Signaling and Hypothalamic Alterations under AMYR Blockade.

A. Three main signaling pathways drive POMC transcription in the hypothalamus. AMYR signaling through pERK activation can drive POMC. LepR activation can induce pSTAT3 translocation to the nucleus to then drive POMC transcription and inhibit AgRP. Additionally, LepR and IR share a common signaling pathway to alter POMC and AgRP transcription via activation of IRS-1 and downstream PI3K/Akt/FOXO1 signal transduction. In native states Akt phosphorylation of FOXO1 causes its inactivation and self-translocate to the cytoplasm. This event allows for POMC transcription. In the scenario that FOXO1 remains active, it resumes as a native inhibitor of POMC and promotor for AgRP. **B**. In the case of AMYR antagonism with AC187, LepR, IRS-1 and POMC are significantly altered compared to controls.

5. Conclusion

This study further strengthens our proposal that amylin is a critical neuropeptide had direct effects as well as indirect effects through the regulation of other neuropeptides. The disruption of these peptides, namely insulin or leptin, has been extensively reported to drive disease, thus understanding their interactions and how amylin signaling impact such relationships can shed light on novel biomarkers or even therapeutics to target AD. While we unexpectedly found that chronic AC187 administration increased POMC expression, LepR transcription, and total IRS-1 protein expression, we offer rationale that chronic loss of AMYR signaling initiates compensatory mechanisms that drive the translation and transcription of these proteins, in order to maintain homeostatic metabolic status. Overall, our findings here within Chapter 3 show, for the first time, how AMYR signaling may drive important hypothalamic metabolic signaling that could impact other areas more closely associated with AD (hippocampus, cortex). Using more localized activation and inhibition of hypothalamic and hippocampal amylin circuits will clarify why we observed potent increases of POMC, LepR and IRS-1 under AMYR antagonism, but observed no differences or increases in such peptides under amylin receptor activation.

CHAPTER 4
GENERAL DISCUSSION

Sporadic AD is a complex disease where etiology is not exactly known. Thus, furthering our knowledge about risk factors associated with AD may offer new biomarkers for future therapies. Metabolic hormone dysfunction diseases such as obesity-induced Type II diabetes Mellitus (T2DM), are major risk factors for developing AD (344–346). Importantly, AD and T2DM share multiple commonalties including increased OS and inflammation (181,347), hypometabolism in the CNS (277,348), synaptic transmission dysfunction at pre- and post-synaptic sites (349), cognitive decline and memory loss (36,38,350), brain atrophy (37,351,352) and protein aggregation within the brain (353–356). Importantly, as discussed in Chapter 3, aberrant peripheral metabolic hormone signaling can have detrimental effects on CNS function (357–361). Metabolic signaling dysregulation can impact the brain directly through impaired glucose signaling that leads to decreased ATP production, increased ROS production and inflammation or through dysregulation of several important metabolic peptides including insulin, leptin and amylin (243,323,362).

A peripherally made hormone, amylin, has both peripheral and central roles in the regulation of metabolic homeostasis as well as extra-metabolic functions that include cognition (138,139,141,148–150). Importantly, these extra-metabolic functions extend to its ability to also regulate pathogenic events, including oxidative stress resistance(148), possible microglial regulation in inflammatory events [33], Aβ degradation [34], and more reducing Aβ pathology (148–150). However, how amylin and its commonly used analog PRAM, elicits such neuroprotective effects throughout the brain were largely unknown.

In this dissertation I aimed to dissect whether the neuroprotective functions of PRAM therapy in AD mice previously reported by us and others to be important in improving the AD phenotype were driven through the activation of the AMYR within the brain, or rather through peripheral mechanisms that improved metabolic tone and resulted in functional and pathology changes via secondary players (i.e., insulin changes). Secondly, we also set out to survey whether PRAM's effects on cognition and Aβ pathology were mediated through other relevant metabolic neuropeptides that 1) have shown to play an important role in brain neuroprotection and AD, and 2) are known to be associated with or interacts with amylin, specifically in the hypothalamus. These include leptin, insulin, and POMC. Lastly, 3) we aimed to elucidate whether central AMYR inhibition would positively or negatively impact cognition function and amyloid pathologies. This last question is important, given the conflicting reports supporting the use of both AMYR agonist (138,148–150,187) and antagonist as therapies for AD (49,151,165).

First, to address whether improvements in metabolic tone (i.e., reductions in glucose tolerance and increases in insulin sensitivity) could explain the benefits associated with PRAM in our mouse model, we carried out a detailed testing including fasting insulin and glucose, body weight, and insulin and glucose tolerance testing. Our data, however, suggested that chronic PRAM, at the dose given in this study, had no detectable effect on these markers. Thus, we can conclude that PRAM-mediated benefits in AD models cannot be ascribed to overt changes in peripheral metabolic function. These data may be surprising given the known role of PRAM in improving insulin sensitivity clinically [39–43] and reducing weight in leptin resistant states such as obesity [37,38]. However, a plausible explanation here is that we did not detect differences because, unlike the populations in which PRAM is used, there were no alterations in metabolic tone or obese states to begin with. Given the known ability of obesity and diabetic states to accelerate the AD phenotype in AD mouse models (177,325,345,347,365,367) future work will need to examine whether PRAM treatment has an impact on such endpoints under metabolic stress and whether normalization of these endpoints is involved in altering such AD phenotype acceleration.

This work, albeit to a lesser extent, confirms both our previous cognitive and pathology findings in this mouse model. One of the major pitfalls of this study is that we used a shorter treatment design (2 months) and started this work in younger animals compared to Patrick et al., (2019) in which animals were treated for 3 months and tested at 9 months of age [28]. This restricted our ability to detect significant differences primarily only in females, which are known to show an accelerated phenotype compared to male mice of the same strain.

Despite the above procedural limitations and of note, this study was able to detect significant increases in AD pathology (soluble $A\beta_{1\text{-}42}$) when the AMYR was blocked using the AC187 antagonism, increases that were, at least, normalized by PRAM. These findings are of key significance to the field given the current conflict in the literature reporting that both agonism and antagonism reduce pathology. Our data demonstrates that AMYR antagonism fails to reduce pathology while AMYR agonism does. In fact, animals treated with both AC187 and PRAM showed lower levels of soluble $A\beta_{1\text{-}42}$ that animals treated with AC187 alone suggesting that AC187 blockade is amyloidogenic.

One interesting aspect of these data is that PRAM reduced AC187-mediated increases in pathology while being delivered peripherally. At face value, one could speculate that PRAM could be mediating such effects either 1) regulating $A\beta$ processing machinery at a peripheral level 2) that PRAM could be reducing pathology through regulating peripheral metabolic endpoints or 3) by regulating secondary metabolic hormones that in turn drive such reductions in pathology. In relation to the first assertion, to address this in more detail we evaluated the activity of α- , β-, and γ-secretases that cleave APP and lead to the production of $A\beta$ fragments that fibrilize ($A\beta_{1-42}$) or that are cleared or tend not to fibrilize ($A\beta_{1-40}$). Within this study we reported no differences in $CTF\beta$ or $CTF\alpha$ due to treatment in female cortex or hippocampus tissue. This was an unexcepted finding as we have previously reported that PRAM increased hippocampal protein expression of both ADAM10 and BACE1 in APP/PS1 mice [28]. Others [32] , however, have reported that BACE1 activity was not altered by PRAM or human amylin. Thus, our findings, in conjunction with Zhu et al [32], conclude that PRAM may not regulate $A\beta$ pathology through BACE1-related mechanisms. Importantly, we also did not detect changes in activity of these enzymes under AC187 treatment, thus suggesting that APP processing may not be a target associated with AMYR regulation. However, whether peripheral administration of PRAM can drive efflux of $A\beta$ from the CNS outward is an intriguing question that has been alluded to *in vitro* [332] and that should be pursued. In relation to trafficking, we found that increases in plaque-like $A\beta$ was accompanied by a reduced SDS- soluble $A\beta$ fraction when comparing the fraction percentage over total $A\beta_{1-42}$. It is generally agreed upon that SDS, detergent soluble fractions represent any $A\beta$ that is bound to lipid membrane or vesicles, we hypothesize that amylin signaling may regulate pathology through changing the availability of APP at the membrane. Potentially analyzing the SDS-soluble fraction using NMR spectrometry or HPLC methodologies could help annotate what $A\beta_{1-42}$ comprises in this subcellular fraction.

Another potential explanation for our findings is that PRAM, despite being delivered in the periphery, at the doses given, crosses the BBB and outcompetes AC187. The PRAM dose used was shown to be maximally therapeutic in humans and has also been shown to be effective at improving cognitive function and reduce pathology [29]. The AC187 dose used within this study is comparable to doses used in [29,36,37]. However, very little is known about the kinetics of these two molecules *in vivo* when delivered together. Therefore, more detailed pharmacological work will need to be carried out to address this aspect as well.

In relation to our second point, we know that PRAM effects are unlikely to be mediated through altering insulin sensitivity or metabolic activity given our metabolic endpoint phenotyping results. We cannot exclude other peripheral changes such as changes in the microbiome, known to regulate AD pathology (368), could drive such events. Given the role of PRAM in gastric bypass and absorption this has some basis for future studies.

Lastly, in relation to the third plausible mechanism driving changes in pathology, peptides like leptin, insulin, and POMC have been reported to play a role in hippocampal-related learning and memory and are known to interact with amylin receptor signaling. Unfortunately, our profiling of changes in such metabolic peptides, their receptors, or their signaling also did not yield much in terms of clear mechanistic guidance. This is however mitigated by the novel finding that PRAM treatment increased POMC protein expression in the hippocampus. Recently, a α-MSH/MC4R microcircuit has been discovered in the hippocampus which describes that MC4R activation increases LTP and decreased Aβ plaque burden potentially through an increased glial response in APP/PS1 mice [38,39]. Given our findings and recent reports linking between POMC to AD, this aspect should be further explored in future studies; in particular, how amylin may mediate this microcircuit or whether such mechanism is initiated locally within the hippocampus versus the hypothalamus.

Within Chapter 3 we turned to the hypothalamus to better understand AMYR signaling in AD pathogenesis for two main reasons: 1) to determine if AMYR activation/inhibition altered hypothalamic signaling to explain findings from Chapter 2 and 2) to further characterize amylin signaling cascades in the hypothalamus, which may lead to potential novel targets and areas of exploration in the AD field. Again however, significant differences across treatment groups were sparse in relation to AMYR agonism under peripheral PRAM treatment. This may simply reflect a floor effect since APP/PS1 at this age do not have metabolic impairments. However, a rather striking finding was that central AMYR blockade with AC187 increased, POMC expression. Why AMYR agonism through PRAM treatment would increase POMC levels in the hippocampus while AMYR antagonism would do the same in the hypothalamus, at this point is completely unknown. We offer the hypothesis that the chronic blocking of amylin signaling AC187 may have driven a compensatory signaling to increase POMC expression in order to maintain metabolic homeostasis. In parallel to these findings, we also identified that IRS-1 transcription was also increased by AC187, further reflecting compensatory changes. However, at this point, we cannot determine that this is the case. Future work addressing LepR or IR signaling cascades such as the activation of IRS-1/PI3K/Akt/FOXO1 dependent pathways may provide a clearer connection between these findings.

Within this study we also where able to conclude that PRAM activation of AMYR was able to rescue spatial memory impairments. Both mice treated groups with AMYR antagonist were unable to learn the RAWM task. Unlike the impact AC187 had on Aβ pathology, we did not find that AC187 worsened cognition or memory formation compared to AD controls. This may be due to a floor effect where mice are unable to perform any worse at the task than AD controls. Interestingly, however, the early immediate gene, Arc, transcription was driven PRAM in the hippocampus, this was observed *in vivo* and also picked up by RNAseq in our male cohort. Arc plays a role in both synaptic plasticity and long-term memory formation [40,41], as well as $A\beta$ pathology [42] through mediation of endosomal trafficking. While increased Arc has been suggested to drive $A\beta$-related pathologies in AD models [43], we interestingly do not see this phenotype in our experimental paradigm. Given the relationship of Arc to gamma-secretase and presenilin, and our findings showing changes in SDS fraction trafficking and outstanding area of study is to deepen our understanding of Arc signaling in relation to native amyloid trafficking under non-diseased states. We hypothesize that perhaps PRAM may be carrying out such a role. Alternatively, it is plausible that increased Arc does drive $A\beta$ pathology in APP/PS1 mice, however amylin may mediate other compensatory mechanisms to combat this effect, i.e., $A\beta$ efflux or microglia degradation, yet drive improvements in cognition through an Arc related mechanism.

Lastly, in order to expand our ability to find targets that could explain how PRAM drives benefits, we explored the effects of PRAM on the hippocampal transcriptome. Overall, the number of that showed to be significantly differentially expressed was small. This is not entirely unexpected given the chronic nature of our treatment. Another notable aspect was the fact that the genes that were altered in males and females where different. This could simply reflect the different stage of disease at which the transcriptome was sequenced. However, these findings underscore the need to carryout experimental work that is powered to determine differences in males and females independently. Overall, the main take home conclusion of this work was that the genes that were differentially altered by PRAM where all associated with beneficial effects, not negative effects. Thus, based on these data, the likelihood that AMYR activation drives AD

pathogenesis is low. In females, genes that were normalized to WT levels by PRAM were

centered around DNA repair and mitochondrial function and oxidative stress protection, all

aspects known to be altered in AD (162,181,369–371) or regulated by amylin/pram (148). In

males, the main genes that were normalized centered around cellular membrane stabilization, and

interestingly showed Arc as one of them. These could speak to our SDS findings and the need to

delve deeper into the membrane dynamics including exosome release, autophagy etc.

In conclusion our work supports the benefits of AMYR activation in AD therapy and does not

support such benefits being ascribed to AMYR antagonism, at least using AC187. Our work

also highlighted some novel mechanisms including those involving POMC signaling as potential

mediators of cognitive improvement and reductions in AD pathology that should be pursued in

future studies. Importantly, we also highlight the relevance of the immediate early gene Arc in

our findings. This is particularly relevant in the context of cognition but also given our soluble

amyloid-beta fraction results and our RNAseq data.

The interpretation of our data is complicated by the fact that the AMYR antagonist was

delivered in the ventricle rather than the hippocampus or they hypothalamus, the two areas that

we investigated in this dissertation. This makes our ability to dissect circuitry very difficult. Our

choice of delivering PRAM peripherally was primarily chosen to be able to address whether

peripheral metabolic changes were involved in the improvements associated with PRAM

delivery in previous studies (138,148). However, this also complicated our ability to dissect the

kinetics of these drugs on our endpoints. There is very little known about the pharmacology of

the AMYR in vivo, importantly we know little regarding the expression levels of the different

AMYR subunits in the different areas and, even whether they have the same affinity for the ligands that we delivered. Thus, future work will need to address the pharmacology much more closely.

REFERENCES

1. Alzheimer's & Dementia | Alzheimer's Association [Internet]. [cited 2021 Mar 26]. Available from: https://www.alz.org/alzheimer_s_dementia

2. James BD, Leurgans SE, Hebert LE, Scherr PA, Yaffe K, Bennett DA. Contribution of Alzheimer disease to mortality in the United States. Neurology [Internet]. 2014 Aug;82(12):1045–50. Available from: https://n.neurology.org/content/82/12/1045

3. Hardy J. The Amyloid Hypothesis of Alzheimer's Disease: Progress and Problems on the Road to Therapeutics. Science [Internet]. 2002;297(5580). Available from: https://pubmed.ncbi.nlm.nih.gov/12130773/

4. Iqbal K, Liu F, Gong C-X, Grundke-Iqbal I. Tau in Alzheimer Disease and Related Tauopathies. Current Alzheimer Research. 2010 Aug;7(8):656–64.

5. Serrano-Pozo A, Frosch MP, Masliah E, Hyman BT. Neuropathological Alterations in Alzheimer Disease. Cold Spring Harbor Perspectives in Medicine [Internet]. 2011 Aug;1(1):a006189. Available from: http://perspectivesinmedicine.cshlp.org/content/1/1/a006189.full

6. Serpell LC. Alzheimer's amyloid fibrils: structure and assembly. Biochimica et Biophysica Acta (BBA) - Molecular Basis of Disease. 2000 Aug;1502(1):16–30.

7. Mandelkow E, Mandelkow EM. Microtubules and microtubule-associated proteins. Current Opinion in Cell Biology. 1995 Aug;7(1):72–81.

8. Dumont M, Stack C, Elipenahli C, Jainuddin S, Gerges M, Starkova NN, et al. Behavioral deficit, oxidative stress, and mitochondrial dysfunction precede tau pathology in P301S transgenic mice. The FASEB Journal [Internet]. 2011 Aug;25(11):4063–72. Available from: www.fasebj.org

9. Desai MK, Sudol KL, Janelsins MC, Mastrangelo MA, Frazer ME, Bowers WJ. Triple-transgenic Alzheimer's disease mice exhibit region-specific abnormalities in brain myelination patterns prior to appearance of amyloid and tau pathology. GLIA [Internet]. 2009 Aug;57(1):54–65. Available from: https://onlinelibrary.wiley.com/doi/full/10.1002/glia.20734

10. Zuo L, Hemmelgarn BT, Chuang CC, Best TM. The Role of Oxidative Stress-Induced Epigenetic Alterations in Amyloid-β Production in Alzheimer's Disease. Oxidative Medicine and Cellular Longevity. 2015;2015.

11. Braak H, Braak E. Frequency of Stages of Alzheimer-Related Lesions in Different Age Categories. Neurobiology of Aging. 1997 Aug;18(4):351–7.

12. FastStats - Leading Causes of Death [Internet]. [cited 2021 Mar 26]. Available from: https://www.cdc.gov/nchs/fastats/leading-causes-of-death.htm

13. Bertram L, Tanzi RE. Genome-wide association studies in Alzheimer's disease. Human Molecular Genetics [Internet]. 2009 Aug;18(R2):R137–45. Available from: https://academic.oup.com/hmg/article/18/R2/R137/606164

14. Jellinger KA, Paulus W, Wrocklage C, Litvan I. Traumatic brain injury as a risk factor for Alzheimer disease. Comparison of two retrospective autopsy cohorts with evaluation of ApoE genotype. BMC Neurology 2001 1:1 [Internet]. 2001 Aug;1(1):1–4. Available from: https://bmcneurol.biomedcentral.com/articles/10.1186/1471-2377-1-3

15. Mayeux R, Stern Y, Ottman R, Tatemichi TK, Tang M-X, Maestre G, et al. The apolipoprotein ε4 allele in patients with Alzheimer's disease. Annals of Neurology [Internet]. 1993 Aug;34(5):752–4. Available from: https://onlinelibrary.wiley.com/doi/full/10.1002/ana.410340527

16. O'Meara ES, Kukull WA, Sheppard L, Bowen JD, McCormick WC, Teri L, et al. Head injury and risk of Alzheimer's disease by apolipoprotein E genotype. American Journal of Epidemiology. 1997 Aug;146(5):373–84.

17. Martin WJ, Martin J. Stealth Adapted Viruses-Possible Drivers of Major Neuropsychiatric Illnesses Including Alzheimer's Disease. 2015; Available from: http://medcraveonline.com

18. Wozniak MA, Shipley SJ, Combrinck M, Wilcock GK, Itzhaki RF. Productive herpes simplex virus in brain of elderly normal subjects and Alzheimer's disease patients. Journal of Medical Virology [Internet]. 2005 Aug;75(2):300–6. Available from: https://onlinelibrary.wiley.com/doi/full/10.1002/jmv.20271

19. Fulop T, Witkowski JM, Bourgade K, Khalil A, Zerif E, Larbi A, et al. Can an Infection Hypothesis Explain the Beta Amyloid Hypothesis of Alzheimer's Disease? Frontiers in Aging Neuroscience. 2018 Aug;0:224.

20. Soscia SJ, Kirby JE, Washicosky KJ, Tucker SM, Ingelsson M, Hyman B, et al. The Alzheimer's Disease-Associated Amyloid β-Protein Is an Antimicrobial Peptide. PLOS ONE [Internet]. 2010 Aug;5(3):e9505. Available from: https://journals.plos.org/plosone/article?id=10.1371/journal.pone.0009505

21. Gamez P, Caballero AB. Copper in Alzheimer's disease: Implications in amyloid aggregation and neurotoxicity. AIP Advances [Internet]. 2015 Aug;5(9):92503. Available from: https://aip.scitation.org/doi/abs/10.1063/1.4921314

22. Curtain CC, Ali F, Volitakis I, Cherny RA, Norton RS, Beyreuther K, et al. Alzheimer's Disease Amyloid-β Binds Copper and Zinc to Generate an Allosterically Ordered Membrane-penetrating Structure Containing Superoxide Dismutase-like Subunits *. Journal of Biological Chemistry [Internet]. 2001 Aug;276(23):20466–73. Available from: http://www.jbc.org/article/S0021925819404973/fulltext

23. Evans DA, Hebert LE, Beckett LA, Scherr PA, Albert MS, Chown MJ, et al. Education and Other Measures of Socioeconomic Status and Risk of Incident Alzheimer Disease in a Defined Population of Older Persons. Archives of Neurology [Internet]. 1997 Aug;54(11):1399–405. Available from: https://jamanetwork.com/journals/jamaneurology/fullarticle/594800

24. Whitmer R, Gunderson E, Quesenberry C, Zhou J, Yaffe K. Body Mass Index in Midlife and Risk of Alzheimer Disease and Vascular Dementia. Current Alzheimer Research [Internet]. 2007;4(2). Available from: https://pubmed.ncbi.nlm.nih.gov/17430231/

25. Whitmer RA, Gunderson EP, Barrett-Connor E, Quesenberry CP, Yaffe K. Obesity in middle age and future risk of dementia: a 27 year longitudinal population based study. BMJ [Internet]. 2005 Aug;330(7504):1360. Available from: https://www.bmj.com/content/330/7504/1360

26. LEIBSON CL, ROCCA WA, HANSON VA, CHA R, KOKMEN E, O'BRIEN PC, et al. The Risk of Dementia among Persons with Diabetes Mellitus: A Population-Based Cohort Study. Annals of the New York Academy of Sciences [Internet]. 1997;826(1 Cerebrovascul). Available from: https://pubmed.ncbi.nlm.nih.gov/9329716/

27. Li X, Song D, Leng SX. Link between type 2 diabetes and Alzheimer's disease: from epidemiology to mechanism and treatment. Clinical Interventions in Aging [Internet]. 2015 Aug;10:549. Available from: /pmc/articles/PMC4360697/

28. Huang C-C, Chung C-M, Leu H-B, Lin L-Y, Chiu C-C, Hsu C-Y, et al. Diabetes Mellitus and the Risk of Alzheimer's Disease: A Nationwide Population-Based Study. PLOS ONE

[Internet]. 2014 Aug;9(1):e87095. Available from:
https://journals.plos.org/plosone/article?id=10.1371/journal.pone.0087095

29. Arvanitakis Z, Wilson RS, Bienias JL, Evans DA, Bennett DA. Diabetes Mellitus and Risk of Alzheimer Disease and Decline in Cognitive Function. Archives of Neurology [Internet]. 2004 Aug;61(5):661–6. Available from:
https://jamanetwork.com/journals/jamaneurology/fullarticle/785863

30. J G, HG L, A C, M P, G C. The therapeutic potential of metabolic hormones in the treatment of age-related cognitive decline and Alzheimer's disease. Nutrition research (New York, NY) [Internet]. 2016 Aug;36(12):1305–15. Available from:
https://pubmed.ncbi.nlm.nih.gov/27923524/

31. Taylor R. Insulin Resistance and Type 2 Diabetes. Diabetes [Internet]. 2012 Aug;61(4):778–9. Available from: https://diabetes.diabetesjournals.org/content/61/4/778

32. Kaneto H, Katakami N, Matsuhisa M, Matsuoka TA. Role of reactive oxygen species in the progression of type 2 diabetes and atherosclerosis. Mediators of Inflammation. 2010;2010.

33. Back SH, Kaufman RJ. Endoplasmic Reticulum Stress and Type 2 Diabetes. http://dx.doi.org/101146/annurev-biochem-072909-095555 [Internet]. 2012 Aug;81:767–93. Available from: https://www.annualreviews.org/doi/abs/10.1146/annurev-biochem-072909-095555

34. Evans JL, Goldfine ID, Maddux BA, Grodsky GM. Are Oxidative Stress–Activated Signaling Pathways Mediators of Insulin Resistance and β-Cell Dysfunction? Diabetes [Internet]. 2003 Aug;52(1):1–8. Available from:
https://diabetes.diabetesjournals.org/content/52/1/1

35. Schwartz RS. Exercise Training in Treatment of Diabetes Mellitus in Elderly Patients. Diabetes Care [Internet]. 1990 Aug;13(Supplement 2):77–85. Available from:
https://care.diabetesjournals.org/content/13/Supplement_2/77

36. Moran C, Beare R, Phan TG, Bruce DG, Callisaya ML, Srikanth V. Type 2 diabetes mellitus and biomarkers of neurodegeneration. Neurology [Internet]. 2015 Aug;85(13):1123–30. Available from: https://n.neurology.org/content/85/13/1123

37. Pérez-González R, Alvira-Botero MX, Robayo O, Antequera D, Garzón M, Martín-Moreno AM, et al. Leptin gene therapy attenuates neuronal damages evoked by amyloid-β and rescues memory deficits in APP/PS1 mice. Gene Therapy 2014 21:3 [Internet]. 2014 Aug;21(3):298–308. Available from: https://www.nature.com/articles/gt201385

38. Wennberg AM v, Spira AP, Pettigrew C, Soldan A, Zipunnikov V, Rebok GW, et al. Blood glucose levels and cortical thinning in cognitively normal, middle-aged adults. Journal of the Neurological Sciences. 2016 Aug;365:89–95.

39. K. Dash S. Cognitive Impairment and Diabetes. Recent Patents on Endocrine, Metabolic & Immune Drug Discovery [Internet]. 2013;7(2). Available from:
https://pubmed.ncbi.nlm.nih.gov/23489242/

40. Biessels GJ, Strachan MWJ, Visseren FLJ, Kappelle LJ, Whitmer RA. Dementia and cognitive decline in type 2 diabetes and prediabetic stages: towards targeted interventions. The Lancet Diabetes & Endocrinology [Internet]. 2014;2(3). Available from:
https://pubmed.ncbi.nlm.nih.gov/24622755/

41. Kelley DE, He J, Menshikova E v, Ritov VB. Dysfunction of Mitochondria in Human Skeletal Muscle in Type 2 Diabetes [Internet]. Am Diabetes Assoc. 2944. Available from:
https://diabetes.diabetesjournals.org/content/51/10/2944.short

42.	Mootha VK, Lindgren CM, Eriksson K-F, Subramanian A, Sihag S, Lehar J, et al. PGC-1α-responsive genes involved in oxidative phosphorylation are coordinately downregulated in human diabetes. Nature Genetics 2003 34:3 [Internet]. 2003 Aug;34(3):267–73. Available from: https://www.nature.com/articles/ng1180

43.	Patti ME, Butte AJ, Crunkhorn S, Cusi K, Berria R, Kashyap S, et al. Coordinated reduction of genes of oxidative metabolism in humans with insulin resistance and diabetes: Potential role of PGC1 and NRF1. Proceedings of the National Academy of Sciences [Internet]. 2003 Aug;100(14):8466–71. Available from: https://www.pnas.org/content/100/14/8466

44.	Wieser V, Moschen AR, Tilg H, Hirszfeld ÓL. Inflammation, Cytokines and Insulin Resistance: A Clinical Perspective.

45.	Burgos-Morón, Abad-Jiménez, Marañón, Iannantuoni, Escribano-López, López-Domènech, et al. Relationship Between Oxidative Stress, ER Stress, and Inflammation in Type 2 Diabetes: The Battle Continues. Journal of Clinical Medicine [Internet]. 2019 Aug;8(9):1385. Available from: www.mdpi.com/journal/jcm

46.	Hasnain M, Vieweg WVR, Hollett B. Weight Gain and Glucose Dysregulation with Second-Generation Antipsychotics and Antidepressants: A Review for Primary Care Physicians. https://doi.org/103810/pgm2012072577 [Internet]. 2015 Aug;124(4):154–67. Available from: https://www.tandfonline.com/doi/abs/10.3810/pgm.2012.07.2577

47.	Eizirik DL, Miani M, Cardozo AK. Signalling danger: endoplasmic reticulum stress and the unfolded protein response in pancreatic islet inflammation. Diabetologia 2012 56:2 [Internet]. 2012 Aug;56(2):234–41. Available from: https://link.springer.com/article/10.1007/s00125-012-2762-3

48.	Mousa YM, Abdallah IM, Hwang M, Martin DR, Kaddoumi A. Amylin and pramlintide modulate γ-secretase level and APP processing in lipid rafts. Scientific Reports 2020 10:1 [Internet]. 2020 Aug;10(1):1–14. Available from: https://www.nature.com/articles/s41598-020-60664-5

49.	Soudy R, Kimura R, Patel A, Fu W, Kaur K, Westaway D, et al. Short amylin receptor antagonist peptides improve memory deficits in Alzheimer's disease mouse model. Scientific Reports [Internet]. 2019 Dec 1 [cited 2021 Apr 2];9(1):1–11. Available from: https://www.nature.com/articles/s41598-019-47255-9

50.	Archbold JK, Flanagan JU, Watkins HA, Gingell JJ, Hay DL. Structural insights into RAMP modification of secretin family G protein-coupled receptors: implications for drug development. Trends in Pharmacological Sciences. 2011 Aug;32(10):591–600.

51.	Hay DL, Christopoulos G, Christopoulos A, Sexton PM. Amylin receptors: molecular composition and pharmacology. Biochemical Society Transactions [Internet]. 2004;32(5). Available from: https://pubmed.ncbi.nlm.nih.gov/15494035/

52.	Sexton PM, Paxinos G, Kenney MA, Wookey PJ, Beaumont K. In vitro autoradiographic localization of amylin binding sites in rat brain. Neuroscience [Internet]. 1994;62(2). Available from: https://pubmed.ncbi.nlm.nih.gov/7830897/

53.	Naot D, Cornish J. The role of peptides and receptors of the calcitonin family in the regulation of bone metabolism. Bone. 2008 Aug;43(5):813–8.

54.	P W, C W, E W, K S. A novel peptide in the calcitonin gene related peptide family as an amyloid fibril protein in the endocrine pancreas. Biochemical and biophysical research communications [Internet]. 1986 Aug;140(3):827–31. Available from: https://pubmed.ncbi.nlm.nih.gov/3535798/

55. Sanke T, Hanabusa T, Nakano Y, Oki C, Okai K, Nishimura S, et al. Plasma islet amyloid polypeptide (Amylin) levels and their responses to oral glucose in Type 2 (non-insulin-dependent) diabetic patients. Diabetologia 1991 34:2 [Internet]. 1991 Aug;34(2):129–32. Available from: https://link.springer.com/article/10.1007/BF00500385

56. Young A, Pittner R, Gedulin B, Vine W, Rink T. Amylin regulation of carbohydrate metabolism. Biochemical Society Transactions [Internet]. 1995;23(2). Available from: https://pubmed.ncbi.nlm.nih.gov/7672355/

57. Young A. Inhibition of Food Intake. Amylin: Physiology and Pharmacology [Internet]. 2005; Available from: https://pubmed.ncbi.nlm.nih.gov/16492542/

58. Gedulin BR, Rink TJ, Young AA. Dose-response for glucagonostatic effect of amylin in rats. Metabolism. 1997 Aug;46(1):67–70.

59. Reidelberger RD, Kelsey L, Heimann D. Effects of amylin-related peptides on food intake, meal patterns, and gastric emptying in rats. https://doi.org/101152/ajpregu005972001 [Internet]. 2002;282(5 51-5):1395–404. Available from: https://journals.physiology.org/doi/abs/10.1152/ajpregu.00597.2001

60. Wang Z-L, Bennet WM, Ghatei MA, Byfield PGH, Smith DM, Bloom SR. Influence of Islet Amyloid Polypeptide and the 8–37 Fragment of Islet Amyloid Polypeptide on Insulin Release From Perifused Rat Islets. Diabetes [Internet]. 1993 Aug;42(2):330–5. Available from: https://diabetes.diabetesjournals.org/content/42/2/330

61. Gedulin BR, Rink TJ, Young AA. Dose-response for glucagonostatic effect of amylin in rats. Metabolism. 1997 Aug;46(1):67–70.

62. Reidelberger RD, Kelsey L, Heimann D. Effects of amylin-related peptides on food intake, meal patterns, and gastric emptying in rats. https://doi.org/101152/ajpregu005972001 [Internet]. 2002;282(5 51-5):1395–404. Available from: https://journals.physiology.org/doi/abs/10.1152/ajpregu.00597.2001

63. Chance WT, Balasubramaniam A, Zhang FS, Wimalawansa SJ, Fischer JE. Anorexia following the intrahypothalamic administration of amylin. Brain Research [Internet]. 1991;539(2). Available from: https://pubmed.ncbi.nlm.nih.gov/1675913/

64. Mesaros A, Koralov SB, Rother E, Wunderlich FT, Ernst MB, Barsh GS, et al. Activation of Stat3 Signaling in AgRP Neurons Promotes Locomotor Activity. Cell Metabolism. 2008 Aug;7(3):236–48.

65. Turek VF, Trevaskis JL, Levin BE, Dunn-Meynell AA, Irani B, Gu G, et al. Mechanisms of Amylin/Leptin Synergy in Rodent Models. Endocrinology [Internet]. 2010 Aug;151(1):143–52. Available from: https://academic.oup.com/endo/article/151/1/143/2456068

66. Olsson M, Herrington MK, Reidelberger RD, Permert J, Arnelo U. Comparison of the effects of chronic central administration and chronic peripheral administration of islet amyloid polypeptide on food intake and meal pattern in the rat. Peptides [Internet]. 2007;28(7). Available from: https://pubmed.ncbi.nlm.nih.gov/17614161/

67. Mollet A, Meier S, Riediger T, Lutz TA. Histamine H1 receptors in the ventromedial hypothalamus mediate the anorectic action of the pancreatic hormone amylin. Peptides [Internet]. 2003;24(1). Available from: https://pubmed.ncbi.nlm.nih.gov/12576097/

68. Gebre-Medhin S, Mulder H, Pekny M, Westermark G, Törnell J, Westermark P, et al. Increased Insulin Secretion and Glucose Tolerance in Mice Lacking Islet Amyloid Polypeptide (Amylin). Biochemical and Biophysical Research Communications. 1998 Aug;250(2):271–7.

69. Christopoulos G, Perry KJ, Morfis M, Tilakaratne N, Gao Y, Fraser NJ, et al. Multiple Amylin Receptors Arise from Receptor Activity-Modifying Protein Interaction with the Calcitonin Receptor Gene Product. Molecular Pharmacology [Internet]. 1999;56(1). Available from: https://pubmed.ncbi.nlm.nih.gov/10385705/

70. Barwell J, Wootten D, Simms J, Hay DL, Poyner DR. RAMPs and CGRP Receptors. Advances in Experimental Medicine and Biology [Internet]. 2012;744:13–24. Available from: https://link.springer.com/chapter/10.1007/978-1-4614-2364-5_2

71. Muff R, Bühlmann N, Fischer JA, Born W. An Amylin Receptor Is Revealed Following Co-Transfection of a Calcitonin Receptor with Receptor Activity Modifying Proteins-1 or -3. Endocrinology [Internet]. 1999 Aug;140(6):2924–7. Available from: https://academic.oup.com/endo/article/140/6/2924/2991037

72. LEUTHÄUSER K, GUJER R, ALDECOA A, McKINNEY RA, MUFF R, FISCHER JA, et al. Receptor-activity-modifying protein 1 forms heterodimers with two G-protein-coupled receptors to define ligand recognition. Biochemical Journal [Internet]. 2000 Aug;351(2):347–51. Available from: /biochemj/article/351/2/347/38388/Receptor-activity-modifying-protein-1-forms

73. Hay DL, Christopoulos G, Christopoulos A, Sexton PM. Determinants of BIBN4096BS affinity for CGRP and amylin receptors; the role of RAMP1. Molecular Pharmacology Fast Forward. 2006;

74. J BKMAT. High affinity amylin binding sites in rat brain. Molecular pharmacology [Internet]. 2019;44(3). Available from: https://pubmed.ncbi.nlm.nih.gov/8396712/

75. Hilton JM, Chai SY, Sexton PM. In vitro autoradiographic localization of the calcitonin receptor isoforms, C1a and C1b, in rat brain. Neuroscience. 1995 Aug;69(4):1223–37.

76. Poyner DR. International Union of Pharmacology. XXXII. The Mammalian Calcitonin Gene-Related Peptides, Adrenomedullin, Amylin, and Calcitonin Receptors. Pharmacological Reviews [Internet]. 2002;54(2). Available from: https://pharmrev.aspetjournals.org/content/54/2/233?ijkey=5c8046175ef3dc6adf3fdc0d33 4a37d8ac8b8182&keytype2=tf_ipsecsha#ref-106

77. Husmann K, Sexton PM, Fischer JA, Born W. Mouse receptor-activity-modifying proteins 1, -2 and -3: amino acid sequence, expression and function. Molecular and Cellular Endocrinology. 2000 Aug;162(1–2):35–43.

78. Christopoulos G, Sexton PM, Paxinos G, Huang X-F, Beaumont K, Toga AW. Comparative distribution off receptors for amylin and the related peptides calcitonin gene related peptide and calcitonin in rat and monkey brain. Canadian Journal of Physiology and Pharmacology [Internet]. 1995;73(7). Available from: https://pubmed.ncbi.nlm.nih.gov/8846397/

79. Flahaut M, Rossier BC, Firsov D. Respective Roles of Calcitonin Receptor-like Receptor (CRLR) and Receptor Activity-modifying Proteins (RAMP) in Cell Surface Expression of CRLR/RAMP Heterodimeric Receptors *. Journal of Biological Chemistry [Internet]. 2002 Aug;277(17):14731–7. Available from: http://www.jbc.org/article/S0021925819608550/fulltext

80. Bhogal R, Smith DM, Bloom SR. Investigation and characterization of binding sites for islet amyloid polypeptide in rat membranes. Endocrinology [Internet]. 1992 Aug;130(2):906–13. Available from: https://academic.oup.com/endo/article/130/2/906/2535870

81. Olgiati VR, Guidobono F, Netti C, Pecile A. Localization of calcitonin binding sites in rat central nervous system: Evidence of its neuroactivity. Brain Research. 1983 Aug;265(2):209–15.

82. Hilton JM, Chai SY, Sexton PM. In vitro autoradiographic localization of the calcitonin receptor isoforms, C1a and C1b, in rat brain. Neuroscience. 1995 Aug;69(4):1223–37.

83. Nakamoto H, Suzuki N, Roy SK. Constitutive expression of a small heat-shock protein confers cellular thermotolerance and thermal protection to the photosynthetic apparatus in cyanobacteria. FEBS Letters. 2000 Aug;483(2–3):169–74.

84. Ueda T, Ugawa S, Saishin Y, Shimada S. Expression of receptor-activity modifying protein (RAMP) mRNAs in the mouse brain. Molecular Brain Research. 2001 Aug;93(1):36–45.

85. Stachniak TJE, Krukoff TL. Receptor Activity Modifying Protein 2 Distribution in the Rat Central Nervous System and Regulation by Changes in Blood Pressure. Journal of Neuroendocrinology [Internet]. 2003 Aug;15(9):840–50. Available from: https://www.onlinelibrary.wiley.com/doi/full/10.1046/j.1365-2826.2003.01064.x

86. Barth SW, Riediger T, Lutz TA, Rechkemmer G. Peripheral amylin activates circumventricular organs expressing calcitonin receptor a/b subtypes and receptor-activity modifying proteins in the rat. Brain Research [Internet]. 2004;997(1). Available from: https://pubmed.ncbi.nlm.nih.gov/14715154/

87. Becskei C, Riediger T, Zünd D, Wookey P, Lutz TA. Immunohistochemical mapping of calcitonin receptors in the adult rat brain. Brain Research. 2004 Aug;1030(2):221–33.

88. Huang C-C, Chung C-M, Leu H-B, Lin L-Y, Chiu C-C, Hsu C-Y, et al. Diabetes Mellitus and the Risk of Alzheimer's Disease: A Nationwide Population-Based Study. Pietropaolo M, editor. PLoS ONE [Internet]. 2014 Jan 29 [cited 2021 Mar 26];9(1):e87095. Available from: https://dx.plos.org/10.1371/journal.pone.0087095

89. Banks WA, Kastin AJ, Maness LM, Huang W, Jaspan JB. Permeability of the blood-brain barrier to amylin. Life Sciences [Internet]. 1995;57(22). Available from: https://pubmed.ncbi.nlm.nih.gov/7475950/

90. le Foll C, Johnson MD, Dunn-Meynell AA, Boyle CN, Lutz TA, Levin BE. Amylin-Induced Central IL-6 Production Enhances Ventromedial Hypothalamic Leptin Signaling. Diabetes [Internet]. 2014;64(5). Available from: https://pubmed.ncbi.nlm.nih.gov/25409701/

91. Mietlicki-Baase EG, Rupprecht LE, Olivos DR, Zimmer DJ, Alter MD, Pierce RC, et al. Amylin Receptor Signaling in the Ventral Tegmental Area is Physiologically Relevant for the Control of Food Intake. Neuropsychopharmacology [Internet]. 2013;38(9). Available from: https://pubmed.ncbi.nlm.nih.gov/23474592/

92. Husmann K, Sexton PM, Fischer JA, Born W. Mouse receptor-activity-modifying proteins 1, -2 and -3: amino acid sequence, expression and function. Molecular and Cellular Endocrinology. 2000 Aug;162(1–2):35–43.

93. Bower RL, Hay DL. Amylin structure-function relationships and receptor pharmacology: implications for amylin mimetic drug development. British Journal of Pharmacology [Internet]. 2016;173(12). Available from: https://pubmed.ncbi.nlm.nih.gov/27061187/

94. Christopoulos A, Christopoulos G, Morfis M, Udawela M, Laburthe M, Couvineau A, et al. Novel Receptor Partners and Function of Receptor Activity-modifying Proteins *. Journal of Biological Chemistry [Internet]. 2003 Aug;278(5):3293–7. Available from: http://www.jbc.org/article/S0021925819309251/fulltext

95. Bailey RJ, Bradley JWI, Poyner DR, Rathbone DL, Hay DL. Functional characterization of two human receptor activity-modifying protein 3 variants. [cited 2021 Mar 26]; Available from: http://spdbv.vital-it.ch/

96. Potes CS, Boyle CN, Wookey PJ, Riediger T, Lutz TA. Involvement of the extracellular signal-regulated kinase 1/2 signaling pathway in amylin's eating inhibitory effect. American Journal of Physiology-Regulatory, Integrative and Comparative Physiology [Internet]. 2012;302(3). Available from: https://pubmed.ncbi.nlm.nih.gov/22129618/

97. Coester B, Pence SW, Arrigoni S, Boyle CN, le Foll C, Lutz TA. RAMP1 and RAMP3 Differentially Control Amylin's Effects on Food Intake, Glucose and Energy Balance in Male and Female Mice. Neuroscience [Internet]. 2020;447. Available from: https://pubmed.ncbi.nlm.nih.gov/31881259/

98. Morfis M, Tilakaratne N, Furness SGB, Christopoulos G, Werry TD, Christopoulos A, et al. Receptor Activity-Modifying Proteins Differentially Modulate the G Protein-Coupling Efficiency of Amylin Receptors. Endocrinology [Internet]. 2008 Aug;149(11):5423–31. Available from: https://academic.oup.com/endo/article/149/11/5423/2455119

99. Dacquin R, Davey RA, Laplace C, Levasseur R, Morris HA, Goldring SR, et al. Amylin inhibits bone resorption while the calcitonin receptor controls bone formation in vivo. Journal of Cell Biology [Internet]. 2004 Aug;164(4):509–14. Available from: http://www.jcb.org/cgi/doi/10.1083/jcb.200312135509

100. Qi R, Luo Y, Ma B, Nussinov R, Wei G. Conformational Distribution and α-Helix to β-Sheet Transition of Human Amylin Fragment Dimer. Biomacromolecules [Internet]. 2013 Aug;15(1):122–31. Available from: https://pubs.acs.org/doi/abs/10.1021/bm401406e

101. Gingell JJ, Burns ER, Hay DL. Activity of Pramlintide, Rat and Human Amylin but not Aβ1–42 at Human Amylin Receptors. Endocrinology [Internet]. 2014;155(1). Available from: https://pubmed.ncbi.nlm.nih.gov/24169554/

102. Hay DL, Garelja ML, Poyner DR, Walker CS. Update on the pharmacology of calcitonin/CGRP family of peptides: IUPHAR Review 25. British Journal of Pharmacology [Internet]. 2018 Aug;175(1):3–17. Available from: https://bpspubs.onlinelibrary.wiley.com/doi/full/10.1111/bph.14075

103. Amylin: Physiology and Pharmacology - Andrew Young - Google Books [Internet]. Available from: https://books.google.com/books?id=25NS2UArEoQC&pg=PA47&source=gbs_toc_r&cad=4#v=onepage&q&f=false

104. Banks WA, Willoughby LM, Thomas DR, Morley JE. Insulin Resistance Syndrome in the Elderly. Diabetes Care [Internet]. 2007 Aug;30(9):2369–73. Available from: https://care.diabetesjournals.org/content/30/9/2369

105. Bailey RJ, Walker CS, Ferner AH, Loomes KM, Prijic G, Halim A, et al. Pharmacological characterization of rat amylin receptors: implications for the identification of amylin receptor subtypes. British Journal of Pharmacology [Internet]. 2012 Aug;166(1):151–67. Available from: https://bpspubs.onlinelibrary.wiley.com/doi/full/10.1111/j.1476-5381.2011.01717.x

106. Lutz TA. Control of food intake and energy expenditure by amylin—therapeutic implications. International Journal of Obesity [Internet]. 2009;33(S1). Available from: https://pubmed.ncbi.nlm.nih.gov/19363503/

107. Trevaskis JL, Parkes DG, Roth JD. Insights into amylin–leptin synergy. Trends in Endocrinology & Metabolism [Internet]. 2010;21(8). Available from: https://pubmed.ncbi.nlm.nih.gov/20413324/

108. Lutz TA, Tschudy S, Mollet A, Geary N, Scharrer E. Dopamine D2 receptors mediate amylin's acute satiety effect. American Journal of Physiology-Regulatory, Integrative and Comparative Physiology [Internet]. 2001;280(6). Available from: https://pubmed.ncbi.nlm.nih.gov/11353673/

109. Roth JD. Amylin and the regulation of appetite and adiposity. Current Opinion in Endocrinology & Diabetes and Obesity [Internet]. 2013;20(1). Available from: https://pubmed.ncbi.nlm.nih.gov/23183359/

110. Geary N. A new way of looking at eating. https://doi.org/101152/ajpregu000662005 [Internet]. 2005 Aug;288(6 57-6). Available from: https://journals.physiology.org/doi/abs/10.1152/ajpregu.00066.2005

111. Mollet A, Gilg S, Riediger T, Lutz TA. Infusion of the amylin antagonist AC 187 into the area postrema increases food intake in rats. Physiology & Behavior [Internet]. 2004;81(1). Available from: https://pubmed.ncbi.nlm.nih.gov/15059694/

112. Gedulin BR, Jodka CM, Herrmann K, Young AA. Role of endogenous amylin in glucagon secretion and gastric emptying in rats demonstrated with the selective antagonist, AC187. Regulatory Peptides. 2006 Aug;137(3):121–7.

113. Rushing PA, Hagan MM, Seeley RJ, Lutz TA, D'Alessio DA, Air EL, et al. Inhibition of Central Amylin Signaling Increases Food Intake and Body Adiposity in Rats. Endocrinology [Internet]. 2001 Aug;142(11):5035–8. Available from: https://academic.oup.com/endo/article/142/11/5035/2989369

114. Clementi G, Valerio C, Emmi I, Prato A, Drago F. Behavioral effects of amylin injected intracerebroventricularly in the rat. Peptides. 1996 Aug;17(4):589–91.

115. Liberini CG, Boyle CN, Cifani C, Venniro M, Hope BT, Lutz TA. Amylin receptor components and the leptin receptor are co-expressed in single rat area postrema neurons. Watanabe M, editor. European Journal of Neuroscience [Internet]. 2016;43(5). Available from: https://pubmed.ncbi.nlm.nih.gov/26750109/

116. Zhang Z, Liu X, Morgan DA, Kuburas A, Thedens DR, Russo AF, et al. Neuronal Receptor Activity–Modifying Protein 1 Promotes Energy Expenditure in Mice. Diabetes [Internet]. 2011 Aug;60(4):1063–71. Available from: https://diabetes.diabetesjournals.org/content/60/4/1063

117. Lutz TA, Coester B, Whiting L, Dunn-Meynell AA, Boyle CN, Bouret SG, et al. Amylin Selectively Signals Onto POMC Neurons in the Arcuate Nucleus of the Hypothalamus. Diabetes [Internet]. 2018;67(5). Available from: https://pubmed.ncbi.nlm.nih.gov/29467172/

118. E BWSWVMJ. Delivery across the blood-brain barrier of antisense directed against amyloid beta: reversal of learning and memory deficits in mice overexpressing amyloid precursor protein. The Journal of pharmacology and experimental therapeutics [Internet]. 2011;297(3). Available from: https://pubmed.ncbi.nlm.nih.gov/11356936/

119. Roth JD, Hughes H, Kendall E, Baron AD, Anderson CM. Antiobesity Effects of the β-Cell Hormone Amylin in Diet-Induced Obese Rats: Effects on Food Intake, Body Weight, Composition, Energy Expenditure, and Gene Expression. Endocrinology [Internet]. 2006;147(12). Available from: https://pubmed.ncbi.nlm.nih.gov/16935845/

120. Mack C, Wilson J, Athanacio J, Reynolds J, Laugero K, Guss S, et al. Pharmacological actions of the peptide hormone amylin in the long-term regulation of food intake, food preference, and body weight. https://doi.org/101152/ajpregu002972007 [Internet]. 2007 Aug;293(5):1855–63. Available from: https://journals.physiology.org/doi/abs/10.1152/ajpregu.00297.2007

121. Riddle M, Frias J, Zhang B, Maier H, Brown C, Lutz K, et al. Pramlintide Improved Glycemic Control and Reduced Weight in Patients With Type 2 Diabetes Using Basal Insulin. Diabetes Care [Internet]. 2007;30(11). Available from: https://pubmed.ncbi.nlm.nih.gov/17698615/

122. Coester B, Koester-Hegmann C, Lutz TA, le Foll C. Amylin/Calcitonin Receptor–Mediated Signaling in POMC Neurons Influences Energy Balance and Locomotor Activity in Chow-Fed Male Mice. Diabetes [Internet]. 2020;69(6). Available from: https://pubmed.ncbi.nlm.nih.gov/32152204/

123. Roth JD, Trevaskis JL, Turek VF, Parkes DG. "Weighing in" on synergy: Preclinical research on neurohormonal anti-obesity combinations. Brain Research [Internet]. 2010;1350. Available from: https://pubmed.ncbi.nlm.nih.gov/20096672/

124. Ernst MB, Wunderlich CM, Hess S, Paehler M, Mesaros A, Koralov SB, et al. Enhanced Stat3 Activation in POMC Neurons Provokes Negative Feedback Inhibition of Leptin and InsulinSignaling in Obesity. Journal of Neuroscience [Internet]. 2009 Sep;29(37):11582–93. Available from: https://www.jneurosci.org/content/29/37/11582

125. Mesaros A, Koralov SB, Rother E, Wunderlich FT, Ernst MB, Barsh GS, et al. Activation of Stat3 Signaling in AgRP Neurons Promotes Locomotor Activity. Cell Metabolism. 2008 Aug;7(3):236–48.

126. Schiöth HB, Chhajlani V, Muceniece R, Klusa V, Wikberg JES. Major pharmacological distinction of the ACTH receptor from other melanocortin receptors. Life Sciences [Internet]. 1996 Aug;59(10):797–801. Available from: https://pubmed.ncbi.nlm.nih.gov/8761313/

127. Adan RAH, Gispen WH. Brain Melanocortin Receptors: From Cloning to Function. Peptides. 1997 Aug;18(8):1279–87.

128. Eiden S, Daniel C, Steinbrueck A, Schmidt I, Simon E. Salmon calcitonin – a potent inhibitor of food intake in states of impaired leptin signalling in laboratory rodents. The Journal of Physiology [Internet]. 2002 Aug;541(3):1041–8. Available from: https://physoc.onlinelibrary.wiley.com/doi/full/10.1113/jphysiol.2002.018671

129. GJ C, AC W, A C, RC T, RB S, KB R. Purification and characterization of a peptide from amyloid-rich pancreases of type 2 diabetic patients. Proceedings of the National Academy of Sciences of the United States of America [Internet]. 1987;84(23):8628–32. Available from: https://pubmed.ncbi.nlm.nih.gov/3317417/

130. Westermark P, Wernstedt C, O'Brien TD, Hayden DW, Johnson KH. Islet amyloid in type 2 human diabetes mellitus and adult diabetic cats contains a novel putative polypeptide hormone. The American Journal of Pathology [Internet]. 1987;127(3):414. Available from: /pmc/articles/PMC1899776/?report=abstract

131. Verma N, Ly H, Liu M, Chen J, Zhu H, Chow M, et al. Intraneuronal Amylin Deposition, Peroxidative Membrane Injury and Increased IL-1β Synthesis in Brains of Alzheimer's Disease Patients with Type-2 Diabetes and in Diabetic HIP Rats. Journal of Alzheimer's Disease [Internet]. 2016;53(1). Available from: https://pubmed.ncbi.nlm.nih.gov/27163815/

132. Ly H, Verma N, Sharma S, Kotiya D, Despa S, Abner EL, et al. The association of circulating amylin with β-amyloid in familial Alzheimer's disease. Alzheimer's & Dementia: Translational Research & Clinical Interventions [Internet]. 2021 Aug;7(1):e12130. Available from: https://alz-journals.onlinelibrary.wiley.com/doi/full/10.1002/trc2.12130

133. Jackson K, Barisone GA, Diaz E, Jin L, DeCarli C, Despa F. Amylin deposition in the brain: A second amyloid in Alzheimer disease? Annals of Neurology [Internet]. 2013 Aug;74(4):517–26. Available from: https://onlinelibrary.wiley.com/doi/full/10.1002/ana.23956

134. Lorenzo A, Razzaboni B, Weir GC, Yankner BA. Pancreatic islet cell toxicity of amylin associated with type-2 diabetes mellitus. Nature [Internet]. 1994;368(6473). Available from: https://pubmed.ncbi.nlm.nih.gov/8152488/

135. Bharadwaj P, Solomon T, Sahoo BR, Ignasiak K, Gaskin S, Rowles J, et al. Amylin and beta amyloid proteins interact to form amorphous heterocomplexes with enhanced toxicity in neuronal cells. Scientific Reports 2020 10:1 [Internet]. 2020 Aug;10(1):1–14. Available from: https://www.nature.com/articles/s41598-020-66602-9

136. Lim YA, Ittner LM, Lim YL, Götz J. Human but not rat amylin shares neurotoxic properties with Aβ42 in long-term hippocampal and cortical cultures. FEBS Letters. 2008 Aug;582(15):2188–94.

137. Lim S, Paterson BM, Fodero-Tavoletti MT, O'Keefe GJ, Cappai R, Barnham KJ, et al. A copper radiopharmaceutical for diagnostic imaging of Alzheimer's disease: a bis(thiosemicarbazonato)copper(II) complex that binds to amyloid-β plaques. Chemical Communications [Internet]. 2010 Aug;46(30):5437–9. Available from: https://pubs.rsc.org/en/content/articlehtml/2010/cc/c0cc01175d

138. Adler BL, Yarchoan M, Hwang HM, Louneva N, Blair JA, Palm R, et al. Neuroprotective effects of the amylin analogue pramlintide on Alzheimer's disease pathogenesis and cognition. Neurobiology of Aging. 2014 Apr;35(4):793–801.

139. Qiu WQ, Au R, Zhu H, Wallack M, Liebson E, Li H, et al. Positive Association between Plasma Amylin and Cognition in a Homebound Elderly Population HHS Public Access. J Alzheimers Dis [Internet]. 2014;42(2):555–63. Available from: http://dx.doi.org/10.3233/JAD-140210.

140. Qiu WQ, Zhu H. Amylin and its analogs: A friend or foe for the treatment of Alzheimer's disease? Frontiers in Aging Neuroscience [Internet]. 2014 Jul 29 [cited 2021 Mar 26];6(JUL):186. Available from: www.frontiersin.org

141. Zhu H, Tao Q, Ang TFA, Massaro J, Gan Q, Salim S, et al. Association of Plasma Amylin Concentration With Alzheimer Disease and Brain Structure in Older Adults. JAMA Network Open [Internet]. 2019 Aug;2(8):e199826–e199826. Available from: https://jamanetwork.com/journals/jamanetworkopen/fullarticle/2748598

142. Zhu H, Tao Q, Ang TFA, Massaro J, Gan Q, Salim S, et al. Association of Plasma Amylin Concentration With Alzheimer Disease and Brain Structure in Older Adults. JAMA Network Open [Internet]. 2019 Aug;2(8):e199826–e199826. Available from: https://jamanetwork.com/journals/jamanetworkopen/fullarticle/2748598

143. May PC, Boggs LN, Fuson KS. Neurotoxicity of Human Amylin in Rat Primary Hippocampal Cultures: Similarity to Alzheimer's Disease Amyloid-β Neurotoxicity. Journal of Neurochemistry [Internet]. 1993 Aug;61(6):2330–3. Available from: https://onlinelibrary.wiley.com/doi/full/10.1111/j.1471-4159.1993.tb07480.x

144. Ryan GJ, Jobe LJ, Martin R. Pramlintide in the treatment of type 1 and type 2 diabetes mellitus. Clinical Therapeutics. 2005 Aug;27(10):1500–12.

145. Nyholm B, Ørskov L, Hove KY, Gravholt CH, Møller N, George K, et al. The amylin analog pramlintide improves glycemic control and reduces postprandial glucagon concentrations in patients with type 1 diabetes mellitus. Metabolism. 1999 Aug;48(7):935–41.

146. Riddle M, Pencek R, Charenkavanich S, Lutz K, Wilhelm K, Porter L. Randomized Comparison of Pramlintide or Mealtime Insulin Added to Basal Insulin Treatment for Patients With Type 2 Diabetes. Diabetes Care [Internet]. 2009 Aug;32(9):1577–82. Available from: https://care.diabetesjournals.org/content/32/9/1577

147. Garcia-Alloza M, Robbins EM, Zhang-Nunes SX, Purcell SM, Betensky RA, Raju S, et al. Characterization of amyloid deposition in the APPswe/PS1dE9 mouse model of Alzheimer disease. Neurobiology of Disease. 2006 Aug;24(3):516–24.

148. Patrick S, Corrigan R, Grizzanti J, Mey M, Blair J, Pallas M, et al. Neuroprotective Effects of the Amylin Analog, Pramlintide, on Alzheimer's Disease Are Associated with Oxidative Stress Regulation Mechanisms. Journal of Alzheimer's Disease [Internet]. 2019;69(1). Available from: https://pubmed.ncbi.nlm.nih.gov/30958347/

149. Zhu H, Wang X, Wallack M, Li H, Carreras I, Dedeoglu A, et al. Intraperitoneal injection of the pancreatic peptide amylin potently reduces behavioral impairment and brain amyloid pathology in murine models of Alzheimer's disease. Molecular Psychiatry [Internet]. 2014;20(2). Available from: https://pubmed.ncbi.nlm.nih.gov/24614496/

150. Zhu H, Xue X, Wang E, Wallack M, Na H, Hooker JM, et al. Amylin receptor ligands reduce the pathological cascade of Alzheimer's disease. Neuropharmacology [Internet]. 2017;119. Available from: https://pubmed.ncbi.nlm.nih.gov/28363773/

151. Soudy R, Patel A, Fu W, Kaur K, MacTavish D, Westaway D, et al. Cyclic AC253, a novel amylin receptor antagonist, improves cognitive deficits in a mouse model of Alzheimer's disease. Alzheimer's & Dementia: Translational Research & Clinical Interventions. 2017 Aug;3(1):44–56.

152. Kimura R, Mactavish & D, Yang J, Westaway & D, Jhamandas JH. Pramlintide Antagonizes Beta Amyloid (Aβ)- and Human Amylin-Induced Depression of Hippocampal Long-Term Potentiation. Molecular Neurobiology. 2035;

153. Patel A, Shiritsu S, Tokyo Y, Daigaku R, Fu W, Soudy R, et al. Genetic Depletion of Amylin/Calcitonin Receptors Improves Memory and Learning in Transgenic Alzheimer's Disease Mouse Models. Available from: https://doi.org/10.21203/rs.3.rs-515476/v1

154. Bennett RG, Hamel FG, Duckworth WC. An Insulin-Degrading Enzyme Inhibitor Decreases Amylin Degradation, Increases Amylin-Induced Cytotoxicity, and Increases Amyloid Formation in Insulinoma Cell Cultures. Diabetes [Internet]. 2003 Aug;52(9):2315–20. Available from: https://diabetes.diabetesjournals.org/content/52/9/2315

155. Fu W, Ruangkittisakul A, MacTavish D, Shi JY, Ballanyi K, Jhamandas JH. Amyloid β (Aβ) Peptide Directly Activates Amylin-3 Receptor Subtype by Triggering Multiple Intracellular Signaling Pathways. Journal of Biological Chemistry [Internet]. 2012;287(22). Available from: https://pubmed.ncbi.nlm.nih.gov/22500019/

156. Andreetto E, Yan L-M, Caporale A, Kapurniotu A. Dissecting the Role of Single Regions of an IAPP Mimic and IAPP in Inhibition of Ab40 Amyloid Formation and Cytotoxicity. Available from: http://dx.doi.org/10.1002/cbic.201100192.

157. Tao Q, Zhu H, Chen X, Stern RA, Kowall N, Au R, et al. Pramlintide: The Effects of a Single Drug Injection on Blood Phosphatidylcholine Profile for Alzheimer's Disease. Xia W, editor. Journal of Alzheimer's Disease [Internet]. 2018;62(2). Available from: https://pubmed.ncbi.nlm.nih.gov/29480193/

158. Edvinsson L, Goadsby PJ, Uddman R. Amylin: localization, effects on cerebral arteries and on local cerebral blood flow in the cat. TheScientificWorldJournal. 2001;1:168–80.

159. Martinez-Valbuena I, Valenti-Azcarate R, Amat-Villegas I, Riverol M, Marcilla I, de Andrea CE, et al. Amylin as a potential link between type 2 diabetes and alzheimer disease. Annals of Neurology [Internet]. 2019 Aug;86(4):539–51. Available from: https://onlinelibrary.wiley.com/doi/full/10.1002/ana.25570

160. Cavallucci V, Ferraina C, D'Amelio M. Key Role of Mitochondria in Alzheimer's Disease Synaptic Dysfunction.

161. Yu Q, Du F, Douglas JT, Yu H, Yan SS, Yan SF. Mitochondrial Dysfunction Triggers Synaptic Deficits via Activation of p38 MAP Kinase Signaling in Differentiated Alzheimer's Disease Trans-Mitochondrial Cybrid Cells. Journal of Alzheimer's Disease. 2017 Aug;59(1):223–39.

162. Du H, Guo L, Yan S, Sosunov AA, McKhann GM, Yan SS. Early deficits in synaptic mitochondria in an Alzheimer's disease mouse model. Proceedings of the National Academy of Sciences [Internet]. 2010 Aug;107(43):18670–5. Available from: https://www.pnas.org/content/107/43/18670

163. Miller KE, Sheetz MP. Axonal mitochondrial transport and potential are correlated. Journal of Cell Science [Internet]. 2004 Aug;117(13):2791–804. Available from: http://www.random.org/.

164. Swerdlow RH, Khan SM. The Alzheimer's disease mitochondrial cascade hypothesis: An update. Experimental Neurology. 2009 Aug;218(2):308–15.

165. Fu W, Patel A, Kimura R, Soudy R, Jhamandas JH. Amylin Receptor: A Potential Therapeutic Target for Alzheimer's Disease. Vol. 23, Trends in Molecular Medicine. Elsevier Ltd; 2017. p. 709–20.

166. Wang X, Wang W, Li L, Perry G, gon Lee H, Zhu X. Oxidative stress and mitochondrial dysfunction in Alzheimer's disease. Vol. 1842, Biochimica et Biophysica Acta - Molecular Basis of Disease. Elsevier; 2014. p. 1240–7.

167. Mohamed LA, Zhu H, Mousa YM, Wang E, Qiu WQ, Kaddoumi A. Amylin Enhances Amyloid-β Peptide Brain to Blood Efflux Across the Blood-Brain Barrier. Carro E, editor. Journal of Alzheimer's Disease [Internet]. 2017;56(3). Available from: https://pubmed.ncbi.nlm.nih.gov/28059785/

168. Qiu WQ, Wallack M, Dean M, Liebson E, Mwamburi M, Zhu H. Association between Amylin and Amyloid-β Peptides in Plasma in the Context of Apolipoprotein E4 Allele. Yan R, editor. PLoS ONE [Internet]. 2014;9(2). Available from: https://pubmed.ncbi.nlm.nih.gov/24520345/

169. Qiu WQ, Au R, Zhu H, Wallack M, Liebson E, Li H, et al. Positive Association between Plasma Amylin and Cognition in a Homebound Elderly Population HHS Public Access. J Alzheimers Dis [Internet]. 2014;42(2):555–63. Available from: http://dx.doi.org/10.3233/JAD-140210.

170. Ott A, Stolk RP, van Harskamp F, Pols HAP, Hofman A, Breteler MMB. Diabetes mellitus and the risk of dementia: The Rotterdam Study. Neurology [Internet]. 1999;53(9). Available from: https://pubmed.ncbi.nlm.nih.gov/10599761/

171. Akter K, Lanza EA, Martin SA, Myronyuk N, Rua M, Raffa RB. Diabetes mellitus and Alzheimer's disease: shared pathology and treatment? British Journal of Clinical Pharmacology [Internet]. 2011;71(3). Available from: https://www.ncbi.nlm.nih.gov/pmc/articles/PMC3045545/

172. Akter S, Rahman MM, Abe SK, Sultana P. Prevalence of diabetes and prediabetes and their risk factors among Bangladeshi adults: a nationwide survey. Bulletin of the World Health Organization [Internet]. 2014;92(3). Available from: https://pubmed.ncbi.nlm.nih.gov/24700980/

173. Plum L, Schubert M, Brüning JC. The role of insulin receptor signaling in the brain. Trends in Endocrinology & Metabolism [Internet]. 2005;16(2). Available from: https://pubmed.ncbi.nlm.nih.gov/15734146/

174. Reno CM, Puente EC, Sheng Z, Daphna-Iken D, Bree AJ, Routh VH, et al. Brain GLUT4 Knockout Mice Have Impaired Glucose Tolerance, Decreased Insulin Sensitivity, and Impaired Hypoglycemic Counterregulation. Diabetes [Internet]. 2016;66(3). Available from: https://pubmed.ncbi.nlm.nih.gov/27797912/

175. Oskarsson ME, Paulsson JF, Schultz SW, Ingelsson M, Westermark P, Westermark GT. In Vivo Seeding and Cross-Seeding of Localized Amyloidosis. The American Journal of Pathology [Internet]. 2015;185(3). Available from: https://pubmed.ncbi.nlm.nih.gov/25700985/

176. Götz J, Ittner LM, Lim Y-A. Common features between diabetes mellitus and Alzheimer's disease. Cellular and Molecular Life Sciences [Internet]. 2009;66(8). Available from: https://pubmed.ncbi.nlm.nih.gov/19266159/

177. Takeda S, Sato N, Uchio-Yamada K, Sawada K, Kunieda T, Takeuchi D, et al. Diabetes-accelerated memory dysfunction via cerebrovascular inflammation and Aβ deposition in an Alzheimer mouse model with diabetes. Proceedings of the National Academy of Sciences of the United States of America. 2010 Apr 13;107(15):7036–41.

178. Reddy VP, Zhu X, Perry G, Smith MA. Oxidative Stress in Diabetes and Alzheimer's Disease. Bierhaus A, editor. Journal of Alzheimer's Disease [Internet]. 2009;16(4). Available from: https://www.ncbi.nlm.nih.gov/pmc/articles/PMC2765716/

179. Münch G, Schinzel R, Loske C, Wong A, Durany N, Li JJ, et al. Alzheimer's disease – synergistic effects of glucose deficit, oxidative stress and advanced glycation endproducts. Journal of Neural Transmission [Internet]. 1998;105(4). Available from: https://pubmed.ncbi.nlm.nih.gov/9720973/

180. Baker LD, Cross DJ, Minoshima S, Belongia D, Watson GS, Craft S. Insulin Resistance and Alzheimer-like Reductions in Regional Cerebral Glucose Metabolism for Cognitively Normal Adults With Prediabetes or Early Type 2 Diabetes. Archives of Neurology [Internet]. 2011;68(1). Available from: https://pubmed.ncbi.nlm.nih.gov/20837822/

181. de Felice FG, Ferreira ST. Inflammation, Defective Insulin Signaling, and Mitochondrial Dysfunction as Common Molecular Denominators Connecting Type 2 Diabetes to Alzheimer Disease. Diabetes [Internet]. 2014;63(7). Available from: https://pubmed.ncbi.nlm.nih.gov/24931033/

182. A V, JS L, M C, LA S, DD B, AR Z, et al. Effects of pramlintide, an amylin analogue, on gastric emptying in type 1 and 2 diabetes mellitus. Neurogastroenterology and motility : the official journal of the European Gastrointestinal Motility Society [Internet]. 2002;14(2):123–31. Available from: https://pubmed.ncbi.nlm.nih.gov/11975712/

183. RR K, MR F, K S, B S, RA V, VD C. Amylin and selective glucoregulatory peptide alterations during prolonged exercise. Medicine and science in sports and exercise [Internet]. 2011 Sep;43(8):1451–6. Available from: https://pubmed.ncbi.nlm.nih.gov/21266924/

184. Boyle CN, Lutz TA. Amylinergic control of food intake in lean and obese rodents. Physiology & Behavior [Internet]. 2011;105(1). Available from: https://pubmed.ncbi.nlm.nih.gov/21324327/

185. Mietlicki-Baase EG, Hayes MR. Amylin activates distributed CNS nuclei to control energy balance. Physiology & Behavior [Internet]. 2014;136. Available from: https://pubmed.ncbi.nlm.nih.gov/24480072/

186. Qiu C, Fratiglioni L. Aging without Dementia is Achievable: Current Evidence from Epidemiological Research. Journal of Alzheimer's Disease [Internet]. 2018 Aug;62(3):933–42. Available from: http://www.grg.org

187. E W, H Z, X W, AC G, M W, JK B, et al. Amylin Treatment Reduces Neuroinflammation and Ameliorates Abnormal Patterns of Gene Expression in the Cerebral Cortex of an Alzheimer's Disease Mouse Model. Journal of Alzheimer's disease : JAD [Internet]. 2017;56(1):47–61. Available from: https://pubmed.ncbi.nlm.nih.gov/27911303/

188. Patel A, Shiritsu S, Tokyo Y, Daigaku R, Fu W, Soudy R, et al. Genetic Depletion of Amylin/Calcitonin Receptors Improves Memory and Learning in Transgenic Alzheimer's Disease Mouse Models. Available from: https://doi.org/10.21203/rs.3.rs-515476/v1

189. Lutz TA. Effects of Amylin on Eating and Adiposity. Handbook of Experimental Pharmacology [Internet]. 2011; Available from: https://pubmed.ncbi.nlm.nih.gov/22249817/#affiliation-1

190. Reiner DJ, Mietlicki-Baase EG, Olivos DR, McGrath LE, Zimmer DJ, Koch-Laskowski K, et al. Amylin Acts in the Lateral Dorsal Tegmental Nucleus to Regulate Energy Balance Through Gamma-Aminobutyric Acid Signaling. Biological Psychiatry [Internet]. 2017;82(11). Available from: https://pubmed.ncbi.nlm.nih.gov/28237459/

191. Baisley SK, Baldo BA. Amylin Receptor Signaling in the Nucleus Accumbens Negatively Modulates μ-opioid-Driven Feeding. Neuropsychopharmacology [Internet]. 2014;39(13). Available from: https://pubmed.ncbi.nlm.nih.gov/24957819/

192. Boccia L, Gamakharia S, Coester B, Whiting L, Lutz TA, le Foll C. Amylin brain circuitry. Peptides [Internet]. 2020;132. Available from: https://pubmed.ncbi.nlm.nih.gov/32634450/

193. Zhu H, Tao Q, Ang TFA, Massaro J, Gan Q, Salim S, et al. Association of Plasma Amylin Concentration With Alzheimer Disease and Brain Structure in Older Adults. JAMA Network Open [Internet]. 2019;2(8). Available from: https://pubmed.ncbi.nlm.nih.gov/31433485/

194. Lim YA, Ittner LM, Lim YL, Götz J. Human but not rat amylin shares neurotoxic properties with Aβ42 in long-term hippocampal and cortical cultures. FEBS Letters. 2008 Aug;582(15):2188–94.

195. Ly H, Verma N, Sharma S, Kotiya D, Despa S, Abner EL, et al. The association of circulating amylin with β-amyloid in familial Alzheimer's disease. Alzheimer's & Dementia: Translational Research & Clinical Interventions [Internet]. 2021 Aug;7(1):e12130. Available from: https://alz-journals.onlinelibrary.wiley.com/doi/full/10.1002/trc2.12130

196. Patel A, Shiritsu S, Tokyo Y, Daigaku R, Fu W, Soudy R, et al. Genetic Depletion of Amylin/Calcitonin Receptors Improves Memory and Learning in Transgenic Alzheimer's Disease Mouse Models. Available from: https://doi.org/10.21203/rs.3.rs-515476/v1

197. Watkins HA, Au M, Hay DL. The structure of secretin family GPCR peptide ligands: implications for receptor pharmacology and drug development. Drug Discovery Today. 2012 Aug;17(17–18):1006–14.

198. Hay DL, Christopoulos G, Christopoulos A, Sexton PM. Determinants of BIBN4096BS affinity for CGRP and amylin receptors; the role of RAMP1. Molecular Pharmacology Fast Forward. 2006;

199. Foll C le, Lutz TA. Systemic and Central Amylin, Amylin Receptor Signaling, and Their Physiological and Pathophysiological Roles in Metabolism. Comprehensive Physiology [Internet]. 2020; Available from: https://pubmed.ncbi.nlm.nih.gov/32941692/

200. Stachniak TJE, Krukoff TL. Receptor Activity Modifying Protein 2 Distribution in the Rat Central Nervous System and Regulation by Changes in Blood Pressure. Journal of Neuroendocrinology [Internet]. 2003 Aug;15(9):840–50. Available from: https://www.onlinelibrary.wiley.com/doi/full/10.1046/j.1365-2826.2003.01064.x

201. Husmann K, Sexton PM, Fischer JA, Born W. Mouse receptor-activity-modifying proteins 1, -2 and -3: amino acid sequence, expression and function. Molecular and Cellular Endocrinology. 2000 Aug;162(1–2):35–43.

202. Ueda T, Ugawa S, Saishin Y, Shimada S. Expression of receptor-activity modifying protein (RAMP) mRNAs in the mouse brain. Molecular Brain Research. 2001 Aug;93(1):36–45.

203. Hay DL, Chen S, Lutz TA, Parkes DG, Roth JD. Amylin: Pharmacology, Physiology, and Clinical Potential. Insel PA, editor. Pharmacological Reviews [Internet]. 2015;67(3). Available from: https://pubmed.ncbi.nlm.nih.gov/26071095/

204. Alamed J, Wilcock DM, Diamond DM, Gordon MN, Morgan D. Two-day radial-arm water maze learning and memory task; robust resolution of amyloid-related memory deficits in transgenic mice. Nature Protocols [Internet]. 2006;1(4). Available from: https://pubmed.ncbi.nlm.nih.gov/17487150/

205. Sun Y, Han J, Lin Z, Song L, Wang C, Jia W. Delayed insulin secretion response during an OGTT is associated with an increased risk for incidence of diabetes in NGT subjects. Journal of Diabetes and its Complications. 2016 Sep;30(8):1537–43.

206. OP M, JE A, MR L, DH W. NIH experiment in centralized mouse phenotyping: the Vanderbilt experience and recommendations for evaluating glucose homeostasis in the mouse. American journal of physiology Endocrinology and metabolism [Internet]. 2009 Sep;297(4). Available from: https://pubmed.ncbi.nlm.nih.gov/19638507/

207. S A, AR B, N D, BC F, J P. Evaluating the glucose tolerance test in mice. American journal of physiology Endocrinology and metabolism [Internet]. 2008 Sep;295(6). Available from: https://pubmed.ncbi.nlm.nih.gov/18812462/

208. JE B, ZJ F, AC H-E, AJ K, SJ P, PM J. Metabolic phenotyping guidelines: assessing glucose homeostasis in rodent models. The Journal of endocrinology [Internet]. 2014;222(3):13–25. Available from: https://pubmed.ncbi.nlm.nih.gov/25056117/

209. YB L, JH L, ES P, GY K, CH L. Personalized metabolic profile estimations using oral glucose tolerance tests. Progress in biophysics and molecular biology [Internet]. 2014 Sep;116(1):25–32. Available from: https://pubmed.ncbi.nlm.nih.gov/25157925/

210. JA B, R P, J C, H M, X Z, X W, et al. Luteinizing hormone downregulation but not estrogen replacement improves ovariectomy-associated cognition and spine density loss independently of treatment onset timing. Hormones and behavior [Internet]. 2016 Sep;78:60–6. Available from: https://pubmed.ncbi.nlm.nih.gov/26497249/

211. Head E, Pop V, Vasilevko V, Hill M, Saing T, Sarsoza F, et al. A Two-Year Study with Fibrillar -Amyloid (A) Immunization in Aged Canines: Effects on Cognitive Function and Brain A . Journal of Neuroscience [Internet]. 2008;28(14). Available from: https://www.ncbi.nlm.nih.gov/pmc/articles/PMC6671080/

212. Head E, Pop V, Sarsoza F, Kayed R, Beckett TL, Studzinski CM, et al. Amyloid-β Peptide and Oligomers in the Brain and Cerebrospinal Fluid of Aged Canines. Journal of Alzheimer's Disease [Internet]. 2010;20(2). Available from: https://pubmed.ncbi.nlm.nih.gov/20164551/

213. D K, B L, SL S. HISAT: a fast spliced aligner with low memory requirements. Nature methods [Internet]. 2015 Sep;12(4):357–60. Available from: https://pubmed.ncbi.nlm.nih.gov/25751142/

214. M P, GM P, CM A, TC C, JT M, SL S. StringTie enables improved reconstruction of a transcriptome from RNA-seq reads. Nature biotechnology [Internet]. 2015;33(3):290–5. Available from: https://pubmed.ncbi.nlm.nih.gov/25690850/

215. Plonski N-M, Johnson E, Frederick M, Mercer H, Fraizer G, Meindl R, et al. Automated Isoform Diversity Detector (AIDD): a pipeline for investigating transcriptome diversity of RNA-seq data. 2019 [cited 2021 Mar 29]; Available from: https://doi.org/10.1186/s12859-020-03888-6

216. MI L, W H, S A. Moderated estimation of fold change and dispersion for RNA-seq data with DESeq2. Genome biology [Internet]. 2014 Sep;15(12). Available from: https://pubmed.ncbi.nlm.nih.gov/25516281/

217. Patterson TA, ... EKL-N, undefined 2006. Performance comparison of one-color and two-color platforms within the MicroArray Quality Control (MAQC) project. nature.com [Internet]. 2006; Available from: https://www.nature.com/articles/nbt1242

218. DJ M, GK S. Testing significance relative to a fold-change threshold is a TREAT. Bioinformatics (Oxford, England) [Internet]. 2009 Sep;25(6):765–71. Available from: https://pubmed.ncbi.nlm.nih.gov/19176553/

219. Szklarczyk D, Morris JH, Cook H, Kuhn M, Wyder S, Simonovic M, et al. The STRING database in 2017: quality-controlled protein–protein association networks, made broadly accessible. Nucleic Acids Research [Internet]. 2017;45(Database issue):D362. Available from: /pmc/articles/PMC5210637/

220. Franz M, Lopes CT, Huck G, Dong Y, Sumer O, Bader GD. Cytoscape.js: a graph theory library for visualisation and analysis. Bioinformatics [Internet]. 2016 Sep;32(2):309. Available from: /pmc/articles/PMC4708103/

221. NT D, JH M, J G, LJ J. Cytoscape StringApp: Network Analysis and Visualization of Proteomics Data. Journal of proteome research [Internet]. 2019 Sep;18(2):623–32. Available from: https://pubmed.ncbi.nlm.nih.gov/30450911/

222. F S, M B, N Š, T Š. REVIGO summarizes and visualizes long lists of gene ontology terms. PloS one [Internet]. 2011;6(7). Available from: https://pubmed.ncbi.nlm.nih.gov/21789182/

223. J W, D D, Z S, B Z. WEB-based GEne SeT AnaLysis Toolkit (WebGestalt): update 2013. Nucleic acids research [Internet]. 2013;41(Web Server issue). Available from: https://pubmed.ncbi.nlm.nih.gov/23703215/

224. J R, R I, V V, M K, C T-L, A R, et al. Pathway enrichment analysis and visualization of omics data using g:Profiler, GSEA, Cytoscape and EnrichmentMap. Nature protocols [Internet]. 2019 Sep;14(2):482–517. Available from: https://pubmed.ncbi.nlm.nih.gov/30664679/

225. Huse JT, Pijak DS, Leslie GJ, Lee VM-Y, Doms RW. Maturation and Endosomal Targeting of β-Site Amyloid Precursor Protein-cleaving Enzyme: THE ALZHEIMER'S DISEASE β-SECRETASE *. Journal of Biological Chemistry [Internet]. 2000 Sep;275(43):33729–37. Available from: http://www.jbc.org/article/S0021925820890681/fulltext

226. JD S, G R, J W, S C, N P, D K, et al. Arc/Arg3.1 mediates homeostatic synaptic scaling of AMPA receptors. Neuron [Internet]. 2006 Sep;52(3):475–84. Available from: https://pubmed.ncbi.nlm.nih.gov/17088213/

227. Korb E, Finkbeiner S. Arc in synaptic plasticity: from gene to behavior.

228. S C, JD S, H O, G L, RS P, N P, et al. Arc/Arg3.1 interacts with the endocytic machinery to regulate AMPA receptor trafficking. Neuron [Internet]. 2006 Sep;52(3):445–59. Available from: https://pubmed.ncbi.nlm.nih.gov/17088211/

229. Hollander PA, Levy P, Fineman MS, Maggs DG, Shen LZ, Strobel SA, et al. Pramlintide as an Adjunct to Insulin Therapy Improves Long-Term Glycemic and Weight Control in Patients With Type 2 Diabetes. Diabetes Care [Internet]. 2003 Sep;26(3):784–90. Available from: https://care.diabetesjournals.org/content/26/3/784

230. Steinerman JR, Irizarry M, Scarmeas N, Raju S, Brandt J, Albert M, et al. Distinct Pools of β-Amyloid in Alzheimer Disease–Affected Brain. Archives of Neurology [Internet]. 2008;65(7). Available from: https://pubmed.ncbi.nlm.nih.gov/18625856/

231. Shabestari MH, Meeuwenoord NJ, Filippov Dmitri v, Huber M. Interaction of the amyloid β peptide with sodium dodecyl sulfate as a membrane-mimicking detergent. Journal of Biological Physics [Internet]. 2016;42(3). Available from: https://pubmed.ncbi.nlm.nih.gov/26984615/

232. McDonald JM, Cairns NJ, Taylor-Reinwald L, Holtzman D, Walsh DM. The levels of water-soluble and triton-soluble Aβ are increased in Alzheimer's disease brain. Brain Research [Internet]. 2012;1450. Available from: https://pubmed.ncbi.nlm.nih.gov/22440675/

233. Mousa YM, Abdallah IM, Hwang M, Martin DR, Kaddoumi A. Amylin and pramlintide modulate γ-secretase level and APP processing in lipid rafts. Scientific Reports 2020 10:1 [Internet]. 2020 Aug;10(1):1–14. Available from: https://www.nature.com/articles/s41598-020-60664-5

234. Wu J, Petralia RS, Kurushima H, Patel H, Jung M, Volk L, et al. Arc/Arg3.1 Regulates an Endosomal Pathway Essential for Activity-Dependent β-Amyloid Generation. Cell [Internet]. 2011 Sep;147(3):615. Available from: /pmc/articles/PMC3207263/

235. P W, C W, E W, K S. A novel peptide in the calcitonin gene related peptide family as an amyloid fibril protein in the endocrine pancreas. Biochemical and biophysical research communications [Internet]. 1986 Aug;140(3):827–31. Available from: https://pubmed.ncbi.nlm.nih.gov/3535798/

236. Wang Z-L, Bennet WM, Ghatei MA, Byfield PGH, Smith DM, Bloom SR. Influence of Islet Amyloid Polypeptide and the 8–37 Fragment of Islet Amyloid Polypeptide on Insulin Release From Perifused Rat Islets. Diabetes [Internet]. 1993 Aug;42(2):330–5. Available from: https://diabetes.diabetesjournals.org/content/42/2/330

237. Isaksson B, Wang F, Permert J, Olsson M, Fruin B, Herrington MK, et al. Chronically Administered Islet Amyloid Polypeptide in Rats Serves as an Adiposity Inhibitor and Regulates Energy Homeostasis. Pancreatology [Internet]. 2005;5(1):29–36. Available from: https://www.karger.com/Article/FullText/84488

238. Eiden S, Daniel C, Steinbrueck A, Schmidt I, Simon E. Salmon calcitonin – a potent inhibitor of food intake in states of impaired leptin signalling in laboratory rodents. The Journal of Physiology [Internet]. 2002 Aug;541(3):1041–8. Available from: https://physoc.onlinelibrary.wiley.com/doi/full/10.1113/jphysiol.2002.018671

239. Guo Z, Jiang H, Xu X, Duan W, Mattson MP. Leptin-mediated Cell Survival Signaling in Hippocampal Neurons Mediated by JAK STAT3 and Mitochondrial Stabilization *. Journal of Biological Chemistry [Internet]. 2008 Aug;283(3):1754–63. Available from: http://www.jbc.org/article/S0021925820696715/fulltext

240. Doherty GH, Oldreive C, Harvey J. Neuroprotective actions of leptin on central and peripheral neurons in vitro. Neuroscience. 2008 Aug;154(4):1297–307.

241. Malekizadeh Y, Holiday A, Redfearn D, Ainge JA, Doherty G, Harvey J. A Leptin Fragment Mirrors the Cognitive Enhancing and Neuroprotective Actions of Leptin. Cerebral Cortex [Internet]. 2017 Aug;27(10):4769–82. Available from: https://academic.oup.com/cercor/article/27/10/4769/3056432

242. Doherty GH, Beccano-Kelly D, Yan S du, Gunn-Moore FJ, Harvey J. Leptin prevents hippocampal synaptic disruption and neuronal cell death induced by amyloid β. Neurobiology of Aging [Internet]. 2013;34(1). Available from: https://pubmed.ncbi.nlm.nih.gov/22921154/

243. Greco SJ, Sarkar S, Johnston JM, Zhu X, Su B, Casadesus G, et al. Leptin reduces Alzheimer's disease-related tau phosphorylation in neuronal cells. Biochemical and Biophysical Research Communications. 2008 Aug;376(3):536–41.

244. Fewlass DC, Noboa K, Pi-Sunyer FX, Johnston JM, Yan SD, Tezapsidis N. Obesity-related leptin regulates Alzheimer's Aβ. The FASEB Journal [Internet]. 2004;18(15). Available from: https://pubmed.ncbi.nlm.nih.gov/15576490/

245. Zhao WQ, Townsend M. Insulin resistance and amyloidogenesis as common molecular foundation for type 2 diabetes and Alzheimer's disease. Biochimica et Biophysica Acta (BBA) - Molecular Basis of Disease. 2009 Aug;1792(5):482–96.

246. Baker LD, Cross DJ, Minoshima S, Belongia D, Watson GS, Craft S. Insulin Resistance and Alzheimer-like Reductions in Regional Cerebral Glucose Metabolism for Cognitively Normal Adults With Prediabetes or Early Type 2 Diabetes. Archives of Neurology [Internet]. 2011 Aug;68(1):51–7. Available from: https://jamanetwork.com/journals/jamaneurology/fullarticle/802106

247. Tan KCB, Shiu SWM, Wong Y, Tam X. Serum advanced glycation end products (AGEs) are associated with insulin resistance. Diabetes/Metabolism Research and Reviews [Internet]. 2011 Aug;27(5):488–92. Available from: https://onlinelibrary.wiley.com/doi/full/10.1002/dmrr.1188

248. Ho L, Qin W, Pompl PN, Xiang Z, Wang J, Zhao Z, et al. Diet-induced insulin resistance promotes amyloidosis in a transgenic mouse model of Alzheimer's disease. The FASEB

Journal [Internet]. 2004 Aug;18(7):902–4. Available from:
https://faseb.onlinelibrary.wiley.com/doi/full/10.1096/fj.03-0978fje

249. Shen Y, Tian M, Zheng Y, Gong F, Fu AKY, Ip NY. Stimulation of the Hippocampal POMC/MC4R Circuit Alleviates Synaptic Plasticity Impairment in an Alzheimer's Disease Model. Cell Reports [Internet]. 2016;17(7). Available from: https://pubmed.ncbi.nlm.nih.gov/27829153/

250. Lau JKY, Tian M, Shen Y, Lau S-F, Fu W-Y, Fu AKY, et al. Melanocortin receptor activation alleviates amyloid pathology and glial reactivity in an Alzheimer's disease transgenic mouse model. Scientific Reports 2021 11:1 [Internet]. 2021 Sep;11(1):1–15. Available from: https://www.nature.com/articles/s41598-021-83932-4

251. R I, T Y, E T, H T, T M, K K. Human Mpv17-like protein is localized in peroxisomes and regulates expression of antioxidant enzymes. Biochemical and biophysical research communications [Internet]. 2006 Sep;344(3):948–54. Available from: https://pubmed.ncbi.nlm.nih.gov/16631601/

252. LJM B, IA K, JP S, L W, BT B, JP L, et al. A systematic analysis of Nrf2 pathway activation dynamics during repeated xenobiotic exposure. Archives of toxicology [Internet]. 2019 Sep;93(2):435–51. Available from: https://pubmed.ncbi.nlm.nih.gov/30456486/

253. M TP, J Z, B T, N KJ. Upregulation of Mitochondrial Redox Sensitive Proteins in LPS-Treated Stefin B-Deficient Macrophages. Cells [Internet]. 2019 Sep;8(12). Available from: https://pubmed.ncbi.nlm.nih.gov/31766320/

254. Zhang T, Guan PP, Liu WY, Zhao G, Fang YP, Fu H, et al. Copper stress induces zebrafish central neural system myelin defects via WNT/NOTCH-hoxb5b signaling and pou3f1/fam168a/fam168b DNA methylation. Biochimica et Biophysica Acta (BBA) - Gene Regulatory Mechanisms. 2020 Sep;1863(10):194612.

255. LM S, D S, LM P, BT W, MA S, A M, et al. A PTIP-PA1 subcomplex promotes transcription for IgH class switching independently from the associated MLL3/MLL4 methyltransferase complex. Genes & development [Internet]. 2016 Sep;30(2):149–63. Available from: https://pubmed.ncbi.nlm.nih.gov/26744420/

256. S B-J, J RD, K F, I G, A N, C L, et al. HERC2 coordinates ubiquitin-dependent assembly of DNA repair factors on damaged chromosomes. Nature cell biology [Internet]. 2010;12(1):80–6. Available from: https://pubmed.ncbi.nlm.nih.gov/20023648/

257. Zhou T, Yi F, Wang Z, Guo Q, Liu J, Bai N, et al. The Functions of DNA Damage Factor RNF8 in the Pathogenesis and Progression of Cancer. International Journal of Biological Sciences [Internet]. 2019;15(5):909. Available from: /pmc/articles/PMC6535783/

258. Ogunniyi A, Baiyewu O, Gureje O, Hall KS, Unverzagt F, Siu SH, et al. Epidemiology of dementia in Nigeria: results from the Indianapolis–Ibadan study. European Journal of Neurology [Internet]. 2000 Sep;7(5):485–90. Available from: https://onlinelibrary.wiley.com/doi/full/10.1046/j.1468-1331.2000.00124.x

259. M B-M, P J, A C-T, L Y, D P-M, J Z, et al. Lack of GDAP1 induces neuronal calcium and mitochondrial defects in a knockout mouse model of charcot-marie-tooth neuropathy. PLoS genetics [Internet]. 2015 Sep;11(4). Available from: https://pubmed.ncbi.nlm.nih.gov/25860513/

260. Achari C, Winslow S, Larsson C. Down Regulation of CLDND1 Induces Apoptosis in Breast Cancer Cells. PLOS ONE [Internet]. 2015 Sep;10(6):e0130300. Available from: https://journals.plos.org/plosone/article?id=10.1371/journal.pone.0130300

261. Sural-Fehr T, Bongarzone ER. How membrane dysfunction influences neuronal survival pathways in sphingolipid storage disorders. Journal of neuroscience research [Internet]. 2016 Sep;94(11):1042. Available from: /pmc/articles/PMC5027971/

262. Ambroggio EE, Kim DH, Separovic F, Barrow CJ, Barnham KJ, Bagatolli LA, et al. Surface Behavior and Lipid Interaction of Alzheimer β-Amyloid Peptide 1–42: A Membrane-Disrupting Peptide. Biophysical Journal. 2005 Sep;88(4):2706–13.

263. Lau TL, Ambroggio EE, Tew DJ, Cappai R, Masters CL, Fidelio GD, et al. Amyloid-β Peptide Disruption of Lipid Membranes and the Effect of Metal Ions. Journal of Molecular Biology. 2006 Sep;356(3):759–70.

264. Haughey NJ, Bandaru VVR, Bae M, Mattson MP. Roles for dysfunctional sphingolipid metabolism in Alzheimer's disease neuropathogenesis. Biochimica et Biophysica Acta (BBA) - Molecular and Cell Biology of Lipids. 2010 Sep;1801(8):878–86.

265. CK B, PE S, F K, J A, F S-S, L B, et al. Gain-of-Function Mutations in KCNN3 Encoding the Small-Conductance Ca 2+-Activated K + Channel SK3 Cause Zimmermann-Laband Syndrome. American journal of human genetics [Internet]. 2019 Oct;104(6):1139–57. Available from: https://pubmed.ncbi.nlm.nih.gov/31155282/

266. N Z, S H, L L, D H, Y Y, X D, et al. Suppression of KV7/KCNQ potassium channel enhances neuronal differentiation of PC12 cells. Neuroscience [Internet]. 2016 Oct;333:356–67. Available from: https://pubmed.ncbi.nlm.nih.gov/27450567/

267. Brigidi GS, Santyr B, Shimell J, Jovellar B, Bamji SX. Activity-regulated trafficking of the palmitoyl-acyl transferase DHHC5. Nature Communications 2015 6:1 [Internet]. 2015 Oct;6(1):1–17. Available from: https://www.nature.com/articles/ncomms9200

268. Woodley KT, Collins MO. S-acylated Golga7b stabilises DHHC5 at the plasma membrane to regulate cell adhesion. EMBO reports [Internet]. 2019 Oct;20(10):e47472. Available from: https://onlinelibrary.wiley.com/doi/full/10.15252/embr.201847472

269. PJ K, C W, MM D, BR M, R S, MC B, et al. A ZDHHC5-GOLGA7 Protein Acyltransferase Complex Promotes Nonapoptotic Cell Death. Cell chemical biology [Internet]. 2019 Sep;26(12):1716-1724.e9. Available from: https://pubmed.ncbi.nlm.nih.gov/31631010/

270. Leung H-W, Foo GWQ, VanDongen AMJ. Arc Regulates Transcription of Genes for Plasticity, Excitability and Alzheimer's Disease. bioRxiv [Internet]. 2019 Oct;833988. Available from: https://www.biorxiv.org/content/10.1101/833988v1

271. R B, LL K, M X, GD L, DF Z, T L, et al. The Arc Gene Confers Genetic Susceptibility to Alzheimer's Disease in Han Chinese. Molecular neurobiology [Internet]. 2018 Oct;55(2):1217–26. Available from: https://pubmed.ncbi.nlm.nih.gov/28108859/

272. D G-P, M C, E R, S A, CD N, S W, et al. Distinct beta-arrestin- and G protein-dependent pathways for parathyroid hormone receptor-stimulated ERK1/2 activation. The Journal of biological chemistry [Internet]. 2006 Sep;281(16):10856–64. Available from: https://pubmed.ncbi.nlm.nih.gov/16492667/

273. Porro F, Rosato-Siri M, Leone E, Costessi L, Iaconcig A, Tongiorgi E, et al. β-adducin (Add2) KO mice show synaptic plasticity, motor coordination and behavioral deficits accompanied by changes in the expression and phosphorylation levels of the α- and γ-adducin subunits. Genes, Brain and Behavior [Internet]. 2010 Oct;9(1):84–96. Available from: https://onlinelibrary.wiley.com/doi/full/10.1111/j.1601-183X.2009.00537.x

274. de la Monte SM, Wands JR. Alzheimer's Disease is Type 3 Diabetes—Evidence Reviewed: https://doi.org/101177/193229680800200619 [Internet]. 2008 Sep;2(6):1101–13. Available from: https://journals.sagepub.com/doi/abs/10.1177/193229680800200619

275. Craft S, Asthana S, Cook DG, Baker LD, Cherrier M, Purganan K, et al. Insulin dose–response effects on memory and plasma amyloid precursor protein in Alzheimer's disease: interactions with apolipoprotein E genotype. Psychoneuroendocrinology. 2003 Sep;28(6):809–22.

276. Schubert M, Gautam D, of the … DS-P, undefined 2004. Role for neuronal insulin resistance in neurodegenerative diseases. National Acad Sciences [Internet]. 2004; Available from: https://www.pnas.org/content/101/9/3100.short

277. Hoyer S. Causes and Consequences of Disturbances of Cerebral Glucose Metabolism in Sporadic Alzheimer Disease: Therapeutic Implications. Advances in Experimental Medicine and Biology [Internet]. 2004;541:135–52. Available from: https://link.springer.com/chapter/10.1007/978-1-4419-8969-7_8

278. L M, WH T, K H, A P, A D, G L, et al. Multicenter standardized 18F-FDG PET diagnosis of mild cognitive impairment, Alzheimer's disease, and other dementias. Journal of nuclear medicine : official publication, Society of Nuclear Medicine [Internet]. 2008 Sep;49(3):390–8. Available from: https://pubmed.ncbi.nlm.nih.gov/18287270/

279. A P, MC P, M F, R C, D A, M B, et al. Plasma antioxidants and brain glucose metabolism in elderly subjects with cognitive complaints. European journal of nuclear medicine and molecular imaging [Internet]. 2014;41(4):764–75. Available from: https://pubmed.ncbi.nlm.nih.gov/24297504/

280. Cavallucci V, Ferraina C, D'Amelio M. Key Role of Mitochondria in Alzheimer's Disease Synaptic Dysfunction.

281. Yu Q, Du F, Douglas JT, Yu H, Yan SS, Yan SF. Mitochondrial Dysfunction Triggers Synaptic Deficits via Activation of p38 MAP Kinase Signaling in Differentiated Alzheimer's Disease Trans-Mitochondrial Cybrid Cells. Journal of Alzheimer's Disease. 2017 Aug;59(1):223–39.

282. Du H, Guo L, Yan S, Sosunov AA, McKhann GM, Yan SS. Early deficits in synaptic mitochondria in an Alzheimer's disease mouse model. Proceedings of the National Academy of Sciences [Internet]. 2010 Aug;107(43):18670–5. Available from: https://www.pnas.org/content/107/43/18670

283. Miller KE, Sheetz MP. Axonal mitochondrial transport and potential are correlated. Journal of Cell Science [Internet]. 2004 Aug;117(13):2791–804. Available from: http://www.random.org/.

284. Leibson CL, Rocca WA, Hanson VA, Cha R, Kokmen E, O'Brien PC, et al. Risk of Dementia among Persons with Diabetes Mellitus: A Population-based Cohort Study. American Journal of Epidemiology [Internet]. 1997;145(4). Available from: https://pubmed.ncbi.nlm.nih.gov/9054233/

285. Huang C-C, Chung C-M, Leu H-B, Lin L-Y, Chiu C-C, Hsu C-Y, et al. Diabetes Mellitus and the Risk of Alzheimer's Disease: A Nationwide Population-Based Study. PLOS ONE [Internet]. 2014 Aug;9(1):e87095. Available from: https://journals.plos.org/plosone/article?id=10.1371/journal.pone.0087095

286. Arvanitakis Z, Wilson RS, Bienias JL, Evans DA, Bennett DA. Diabetes Mellitus and Risk of Alzheimer Disease and Decline in Cognitive Function. Archives of Neurology

[Internet]. 2004 Aug;61(5):661–6. Available from:
https://jamanetwork.com/journals/jamaneurology/fullarticle/785863

287. Rodríguez EM, Blázquez JL, Guerra M. The design of barriers in the hypothalamus allows the median eminence and the arcuate nucleus to enjoy private milieus: The former opens to the portal blood and the latter to the cerebrospinal fluid. Peptides. 2010 Sep;31(4):757–76.

288. Myers MG, Olson DP. Central nervous system control of metabolism. Nature 2012 491:7424 [Internet]. 2012 Sep;491(7424):357–63. Available from: https://www.nature.com/articles/nature11705

289. EJ R, A G, N F, R T, JR W, de la Monte SM. Insulin and insulin-like growth factor expression and function deteriorate with progression of Alzheimer's disease: link to brain reductions in acetylcholine. Journal of Alzheimer's disease : JAD [Internet]. 2005;8(3):247–68. Available from: https://pubmed.ncbi.nlm.nih.gov/16340083/

290. TS S, KM B, IA H, ML N, T W-H, J K, et al. Central Nervous System Delivery of Intranasal Insulin: Mechanisms of Uptake and Effects on Cognition. Journal of Alzheimer's disease : JAD [Internet]. 2015 Sep;47(3):715–28. Available from: https://pubmed.ncbi.nlm.nih.gov/26401706/

291. Grillo CA, Piroli GG, Lawrence RC, Wrighten SA, Green AJ, Wilson SP, et al. Hippocampal Insulin Resistance Impairs Spatial Learning and Synaptic Plasticity. Diabetes [Internet]. 2015 Sep;64(11):3927–36. Available from: https://diabetes.diabetesjournals.org/content/64/11/3927

292. Revill P, Moral MA, of Today JRP-D, undefined 2006. Impaired insulin signaling and the pathogenesis of Alzheimer's disease. journals.prous.com [Internet]. Available from: https://journals.prous.com/journals/servlet/xmlxsl/dot/20064212/pdf/dt420785.pdf?p_JournalId=4&p_refId=1032059&p_IsPs=N

293. DJ B, JG S, SL T, SL S, G P, R K, et al. Dysregulation of leptin signaling in Alzheimer disease: evidence for neuronal leptin resistance. Journal of neurochemistry [Internet]. 2014 Sep;128(1):162–72. Available from: https://pubmed.ncbi.nlm.nih.gov/23895348/

294. E U, HW G. Insulin regulates neuronal glucose uptake by promoting translocation of glucose transporter GLUT3. Experimental neurology [Internet]. 2006 Sep;198(1):48–53. Available from: https://pubmed.ncbi.nlm.nih.gov/16337941/

295. E G, M S, E B, AW X, R J, T B, et al. Agouti-related peptide-expressing neurons are mandatory for feeding. Nature neuroscience [Internet]. 2005 Sep;8(10):1289–91. Available from: https://pubmed.ncbi.nlm.nih.gov/16158063/

296. N B, LT D, CE L, J Y, H F, T W, et al. Divergence of melanocortin pathways in the control of food intake and energy expenditure. Cell [Internet]. 2005 Sep;123(3):493–505. Available from: https://pubmed.ncbi.nlm.nih.gov/16269339/

297. Belgardt BF, Husch A, Rother E, metabolism MBE-C, undefined 2008. PDK1 deficiency in POMC-expressing cells reveals FOXO1-dependent and-independent pathways in control of energy homeostasis and stress response. Elsevier [Internet]. Available from: https://www.sciencedirect.com/science/article/pii/S1550413108000077

298. Cao Y, Nakata M, Okamoto S, Takano E, Yada T, Minokoshi Y, et al. PDK1-Foxo1 in agouti-related peptide neurons regulates energy homeostasis by modulating food intake and energy expenditure. PLoS ONE. 2011;6(4).

299. AM B, CS M. Drug Insight: the role of leptin in human physiology and pathophysiology–emerging clinical applications. Nature clinical practice Endocrinology & metabolism

[Internet]. 2006 Sep;2(6):318–27. Available from:
https://pubmed.ncbi.nlm.nih.gov/16932309/

300. E J. Leptin signaling, adiposity, and energy balance. Annals of the New York Academy of Sciences [Internet]. 2002;967:379–88. Available from:
https://pubmed.ncbi.nlm.nih.gov/12079865/

301. N H, DV R, SL J, JR S. Peripherally administered [Nle4,D-Phe7]-alpha-melanocyte stimulating hormone increases resting metabolic rate, while peripheral agouti-related protein has no effect, in wild type C57BL/6 and ob/ob mice. Journal of molecular endocrinology [Internet]. 2004 Sep;33(3):693–703. Available from:
https://pubmed.ncbi.nlm.nih.gov/15591028/

302. Lee DK, Jeong JH, Chun S-K, Jr. SC, Jo Y-H. Interplay between glucose and leptin signalling determines the strength of GABAergic synapses at POMC neurons. Nature Communications 2015 6:1 [Internet]. 2015 Sep;6(1):1–12. Available from:
https://www.nature.com/articles/ncomms7618

303. Pan WW, Myers MG. Leptin and the maintenance of elevated body weight. Nature Reviews Neuroscience 2018 19:2 [Internet]. 2018 Sep;19(2):95–105. Available from:
https://www.nature.com/articles/nrn.2017.168

304. Hill JW, Williams KW, Ye C, of … JL-TJ, undefined 2008. Acute effects of leptin require PI3K signaling in hypothalamic proopiomelanocortin neurons in mice. Am Soc Clin Investig [Internet]. Available from: https://www.jci.org/articles/view/32964

305. Ren H, Orozco IJ, Su Y, Suyama S, Cell RG-J-, undefined 2012. FoxO1 target Gpr17 activates AgRP neurons to regulate food intake. Elsevier [Internet]. Available from:
https://www.sciencedirect.com/science/article/pii/S0092867412005776

306. A K, AC K, JC B. CNS-targets in control of energy and glucose homeostasis. Current opinion in pharmacology [Internet]. 2009 Sep;9(6):794–804. Available from:
https://pubmed.ncbi.nlm.nih.gov/19884043/

307. E R, DK S, MS K. Emerging role of the brain in the homeostatic regulation of energy and glucose metabolism. Experimental & molecular medicine [Internet]. 2016 Sep;48(3). Available from: https://pubmed.ncbi.nlm.nih.gov/26964832/

308. SF L, NJ H, K C. Hypothalamic paraventricular nucleus lesions produce overeating and obesity in the rat. Physiology & behavior [Internet]. 1981;27(6):1031–40. Available from:
https://pubmed.ncbi.nlm.nih.gov/7335803/

309. H K, Y H, H Y. Increase in sympathetic outflow by paraventricular nucleus stimulation in awake rats. The American journal of physiology [Internet]. 1989;256(6 Pt 2). Available from: https://pubmed.ncbi.nlm.nih.gov/2567578/

310. D H, CA L, V F-H, JH D, Q F, LR B, et al. Targeted disruption of the melanocortin-4 receptor results in obesity in mice. Cell [Internet]. 1997 Sep;88(1):131–41. Available from: https://pubmed.ncbi.nlm.nih.gov/9019399/

311. A V-A, JG M, KL E, RC S, EA N, RD C, et al. Role of the central melanocortin circuitry in adaptive thermogenesis of brown adipose tissue. Endocrinology [Internet]. 2007 Sep;148(4):1550–60. Available from: https://pubmed.ncbi.nlm.nih.gov/17194736/

312. BG S, SF L. Neuropeptide Y: stimulation of feeding and drinking by injection into the paraventricular nucleus. Life sciences [Internet]. 1984 Sep;35(26):2635–42. Available from: https://pubmed.ncbi.nlm.nih.gov/6549039/

313. Boyle CN, Lutz TA, le Foll C. Amylin – Its role in the homeostatic and hedonic control of eating and recent developments of amylin analogs to treat obesity. Molecular Metabolism [Internet]. 2018;8. Available from: https://pubmed.ncbi.nlm.nih.gov/29203236/

314. Liberini CG, Borner T, Boyle CN, Lutz TA. The satiating hormone amylin enhances neurogenesis in the area postrema of adult rats. Molecular Metabolism [Internet]. 2016;5(10). Available from: https://pubmed.ncbi.nlm.nih.gov/27688997/

315. Lutz TA. The role of amylin in the control of energy homeostasis. American Journal of Physiology-Regulatory, Integrative and Comparative Physiology [Internet]. 2010;298(6). Available from: https://pubmed.ncbi.nlm.nih.gov/20357016/

316. JW S, JK E, KW W. Neuronal circuits that regulate feeding behavior and metabolism. Trends in neurosciences [Internet]. 2013 Sep;36(9):504–12. Available from: https://pubmed.ncbi.nlm.nih.gov/23790727/

317. Ishii M, Iadecola C. Metabolic and Non-Cognitive Manifestations of Alzheimer's Disease: The Hypothalamus as Both Culprit and Target of Pathology. Cell Metabolism. 2015 Sep;22(5):761–76.

318. ZB A, ZW L, N W, DM E, E B, JM F, et al. UCP2 mediates ghrelin's action on NPY/AgRP neurons by lowering free radicals. Nature [Internet]. 2008 Sep;454(7206):846–51. Available from: https://pubmed.ncbi.nlm.nih.gov/18668043/

319. JP T, CX Y, EA S, SJ G, BH H, MO D, et al. Obesity is associated with hypothalamic injury in rodents and humans. The Journal of clinical investigation [Internet]. 2012 Sep;122(1):153–62. Available from: https://pubmed.ncbi.nlm.nih.gov/22201683/

320. Bracke A, Domanska G, Bracke K, Harzsch S, van den Brandt J, Bröker B, et al. Obesity Impairs Mobility and Adult Hippocampal Neurogenesis. Journal of Experimental Neuroscience [Internet]. 2019;13. Available from: /pmc/articles/PMC6852358/

321. LM Y, RB G, DE D, C S, MT W, CV V, et al. Impairment of cognitive flexibility in type 2 diabetic db/db mice. Behavioural brain research [Internet]. 2019 Sep;371. Available from: https://pubmed.ncbi.nlm.nih.gov/31141724/

322. TJ N, MK S, J H, DL A. Insulin, PKC signaling pathways and synaptic remodeling during memory storage and neuronal repair. European journal of pharmacology [Internet]. 2008 Sep;585(1):76–87. Available from: https://pubmed.ncbi.nlm.nih.gov/18402935/

323. PI M, MS S, C S, R S, CR O. Insulin protects against amyloid beta-peptide toxicity in brain mitochondria of diabetic rats. Neurobiology of disease [Internet]. 2005;18(3):628–37. Available from: https://pubmed.ncbi.nlm.nih.gov/15755688/

324. of neurology SC-A, undefined 2005. Insulin resistance and cognitive impairment: a view through the prism of epidemiology. jamanetwork.com [Internet]. Available from: https://jamanetwork.com/journals/jamaneurology/article-abstract/788821

325. E S, BM T, EJ R, JL C, TR N, R T, et al. Impaired insulin and insulin-like growth factor expression and signaling mechanisms in Alzheimer's disease–is this type 3 diabetes? Journal of Alzheimer's disease : JAD [Internet]. 2005;7(1):63–80. Available from: https://pubmed.ncbi.nlm.nih.gov/15750215/

326. Craft S, Baker LD, Montine TJ, Minoshima S, Watson GS, Claxton A, et al. Intranasal Insulin Therapy for Alzheimer Disease and Amnestic Mild Cognitive Impairment. Archives of Neurology [Internet]. 2012 Sep;69(1):29. Available from: /pmc/articles/PMC3260944/

327. A V, V G, M D, C T, A G, A F, et al. Leptin increases axonal growth cone size in developing mouse cortical neurons by convergent signals inactivating glycogen synthase

kinase-3beta. The Journal of biological chemistry [Internet]. 2006 Sep;281(18):12950–8. Available from: https://pubmed.ncbi.nlm.nih.gov/16522636/

328. JC G, M G, W Z, XY L. Leptin increases adult hippocampal neurogenesis in vivo and in vitro. The Journal of biological chemistry [Internet]. 2008 Sep;283(26):18238–47. Available from: https://pubmed.ncbi.nlm.nih.gov/18367451/

329. Z W, AP S, Y G, S W, F Z, T H, et al. Leptin protects against 6-hydroxydopamine-induced dopaminergic cell death via mitogen-activated protein kinase signaling. The Journal of biological chemistry [Internet]. 2007 Sep;282(47):34479–91. Available from: https://pubmed.ncbi.nlm.nih.gov/17895242/

330. MG M, MA C, H M. Mechanisms of leptin action and leptin resistance. Annual review of physiology [Internet]. 2008;70:537–56. Available from: https://pubmed.ncbi.nlm.nih.gov/17937601/

331. I G, XH M, XM Y, L R, N B. Leptin resistance during aging is independent of fat mass. Diabetes [Internet]. 2002;51(4):1016–21. Available from: https://pubmed.ncbi.nlm.nih.gov/11916920/

332. B B, B S, K S, A P, E S, M G, et al. Adipocytokines and CD34 progenitor cells in Alzheimer's disease. PloS one [Internet]. 2011;6(5). Available from: https://pubmed.ncbi.nlm.nih.gov/21633502/

333. KF H, K L, FA T, C R, TB H, K Y. Serum leptin level and cognition in the elderly: Findings from the Health ABC Study. Neurobiology of aging [Internet]. 2009 Sep;30(9):1483–9. Available from: https://pubmed.ncbi.nlm.nih.gov/18358569/

334. Lieb W. Association of Plasma Leptin Levels With Incident Alzheimer Disease and MRI Measures of Brain Aging. JAMA [Internet]. 2009;302(23). Available from: https://pubmed.ncbi.nlm.nih.gov/20009056/

335. F F, AR S, C P, E M, AR G. Abnormal pro-opiomelanocortin processing in Alzheimer's disease. A case report. Functional Neurology [Internet]. 1987 Sep;2(3):349–53. Available from: https://europepmc.org/article/med/3692276

336. Do K, Laing BT, Landry T, Bunner W, Mersaud N, Matsubara T, et al. The effects of exercise on hypothalamic neurodegeneration of Alzheimer's disease mouse model. PLOS ONE [Internet]. 2018 Sep;13(1):e0190205. Available from: https://journals.plos.org/plosone/article?id=10.1371/journal.pone.0190205

337. Lutz T. Pancreatic Amylin as a Centrally Acting Satiating Hormone. Current Drug Targets [Internet]. 2005;6(2). Available from: https://pubmed.ncbi.nlm.nih.gov/15777188/

338. Riddle M, Pencek R, Charenkavanich S, Lutz K, Wilhelm K, Porter L. Randomized Comparison of Pramlintide or Mealtime Insulin Added to Basal Insulin Treatment for Patients With Type 2 Diabetes. Diabetes Care [Internet]. 2009 Aug;32(9):1577–82. Available from: https://care.diabetesjournals.org/content/32/9/1577

339. Coester B, Koester-Hegmann C, Lutz TA, Foll C le. Amylin/Calcitonin Receptor–Mediated Signaling in POMC Neurons Influences Energy Balance and Locomotor Activity in Chow-Fed Male Mice. Diabetes [Internet]. 2020 Aug;69(6):1110–25. Available from: https://diabetes.diabetesjournals.org/content/69/6/1110

340. le Foll C, Johnson MD, Dunn-Meynell AA, Boyle CN, Lutz TA, Levin BE. Amylin-Induced Central IL-6 Production Enhances Ventromedial Hypothalamic Leptin Signaling. Diabetes [Internet]. 2014;64(5). Available from: https://pubmed.ncbi.nlm.nih.gov/25409701/

341. X X, C C, P G, T Z, S F, J F, et al. Forkhead Box Protein 1 (FoxO1) Inhibits Accelerated β Cell Aging in Pancreas-specific SMAD7 Mutant Mice. The Journal of biological chemistry [Internet]. 2017 Sep;292(8):3456–65. Available from: https://pubmed.ncbi.nlm.nih.gov/28057752/

342. NK R, SS DK, NN H, H A. Understanding the perspectives of forkhead transcription factors in delayed wound healing. Journal of cell communication and signaling [Internet]. 2019 Sep;13(2):151–62. Available from: https://pubmed.ncbi.nlm.nih.gov/30088222/

343. Coester B, Koester-Hegmann C, Lutz TA, Foll C le. Amylin/Calcitonin Receptor–Mediated Signaling in POMC Neurons Influences Energy Balance and Locomotor Activity in Chow-Fed Male Mice. Diabetes [Internet]. 2020 Aug;69(6):1110–25. Available from: https://diabetes.diabetesjournals.org/content/69/6/1110

344. G C, C H, H D, H W. Diabetes as a risk factor for dementia and mild cognitive impairment: a meta-analysis of longitudinal studies. Internal medicine journal [Internet]. 2012 Sep;42(5):484–91. Available from: https://pubmed.ncbi.nlm.nih.gov/22372522/

345. Li X, Song D, Leng SX. Link between type 2 diabetes and Alzheimer's disease: from epidemiology to mechanism and treatment. Clinical Interventions in Aging [Internet]. 2015 Aug;10:549. Available from: /pmc/articles/PMC4360697/

346. Moran C, Beare R, Phan TG, Bruce DG, Callisaya ML, Srikanth V. Type 2 diabetes mellitus and biomarkers of neurodegeneration. Neurology [Internet]. 2015 Aug;85(13):1123–30. Available from: https://n.neurology.org/content/85/13/1123

347. de la Monte SM, Wands JR. Alzheimer's Disease is Type 3 Diabetes—Evidence Reviewed. Journal of Diabetes Science and Technology [Internet]. 2008;2(6). Available from: https://pubmed.ncbi.nlm.nih.gov/19885299/

348. Umegaki H. Type 2 diabetes as a risk factor for cognitive impairment: current insights. Clinical Interventions in Aging [Internet]. 2014; Available from: https://pubmed.ncbi.nlm.nih.gov/25061284/

349. JJ P, L M. Amyloid-beta-induced neuronal dysfunction in Alzheimer's disease: from synapses toward neural networks. Nature neuroscience [Internet]. 2010 Sep;13(7):812–8. Available from: https://pubmed.ncbi.nlm.nih.gov/20581818/

350. Pérez-González R, Alvira-Botero MX, Robayo O, Antequera D, Garzón M, Martín-Moreno AM, et al. Leptin gene therapy attenuates neuronal damages evoked by amyloid-β and rescues memory deficits in APP/PS1 mice. Gene Therapy 2014 21:3 [Internet]. 2014 Aug;21(3):298–308. Available from: https://www.nature.com/articles/gt201385

351. Platt TL, Beckett TL, Kohler K, Niedowicz DM, Murphy MP. Obesity, diabetes, and leptin resistance promote tau pathology in a mouse model of disease. Neuroscience [Internet]. 2016;315. Available from: https://pubmed.ncbi.nlm.nih.gov/26701291/

352. Shen Y, Fu W-Y, Cheng EYL, Fu AKY, Ip NY. Melanocortin-4 Receptor Regulates Hippocampal Synaptic Plasticity through a Protein Kinase A-Dependent Mechanism. Journal of Neuroscience [Internet]. 2013 Aug;33(2):464–72. Available from: https://www.jneurosci.org/content/33/2/464

353. Iqbal K, Liu F, Gong C-X, Grundke-Iqbal I. Tau in Alzheimer Disease and Related Tauopathies. Current Alzheimer Research. 2010 Aug;7(8):656–64.

354. Serrano-Pozo A, Frosch MP, Masliah E, Hyman BT. Neuropathological Alterations in Alzheimer Disease. Cold Spring Harbor Perspectives in Medicine [Internet]. 2011 Aug;1(1):a006189. Available from: http://perspectivesinmedicine.cshlp.org/content/1/1/a006189.full

355. Serpell LC. Alzheimer's amyloid fibrils: structure and assembly. Biochimica et Biophysica Acta (BBA) - Molecular Basis of Disease. 2000 Aug;1502(1):16–30.

356. Mandelkow E, Mandelkow EM. Microtubules and microtubule-associated proteins. Current Opinion in Cell Biology. 1995 Aug;7(1):72–81.

357. Kaneto H, Katakami N, Matsuhisa M, Matsuoka TA. Role of reactive oxygen species in the progression of type 2 diabetes and atherosclerosis. Mediators of Inflammation. 2010;2010.

358. Back SH, Kaufman RJ. Endoplasmic Reticulum Stress and Type 2 Diabetes. http://dx.doi.org/101146/annurev-biochem-072909-095555 [Internet]. 2012 Aug;81:767–93. Available from: https://www.annualreviews.org/doi/abs/10.1146/annurev-biochem-072909-095555

359. Evans JL, Goldfine ID, Maddux BA, Grodsky GM. Are Oxidative Stress–Activated Signaling Pathways Mediators of Insulin Resistance and β-Cell Dysfunction? Diabetes [Internet]. 2003 Aug;52(1):1–8. Available from: https://diabetes.diabetesjournals.org/content/52/1/1

360. Schwartz RS. Exercise Training in Treatment of Diabetes Mellitus in Elderly Patients. Diabetes Care [Internet]. 1990 Aug;13(Supplement 2):77–85. Available from: https://care.diabetesjournals.org/content/13/Supplement_2/77

361. Ward WK, LaCava EC, Paquette TL, Beard JC, Wallum BJ, Porte D. Disproportionate elevation of immunoreactive proinsulin in Type 2 (non-insulin-dependent) diabetes mellitus and in experimental insulin resistance. Diabetologia 1987 30:9 [Internet]. 1987 Aug;30(9):698–702. Available from: https://link.springer.com/article/10.1007/BF00296991

362. Greco SJ, Bryan KJ, Sarkar S, Zhu X, Smith MA, Ashford JW, et al. Leptin Reduces Pathology and Improves Memory in a Transgenic Mouse Model of Alzheimer's Disease. Journal of Alzheimer's Disease. 2010 Aug;19(4):1155–67.

363. Haidar A, Tsoukas MA, Bernier-Twardy S, Yale J-F, Rutkowski J, Bossy A, et al. A Novel Dual-Hormone Insulin-and-Pramlintide Artificial Pancreas for Type 1 Diabetes: A Randomized Controlled Crossover Trial. Diabetes Care [Internet]. 2020 Sep;43(3):597–606. Available from: https://care.diabetesjournals.org/content/43/3/597

364. Cohn C, Berger S, Norton M. Relationship between Meal Size and Frequency and Plasma Insulin Response in Man. Diabetes [Internet]. 1968 Sep;17(2):72–5. Available from: https://diabetes.diabetesjournals.org/content/17/2/72

365. Huajie Li WQQ. Plasma Amylin and Cognition in Diabetes in the Absence and the Presence of Insulin Treatment. Journal of Diabetes & Metabolism [Internet]. 2014;5(11). Available from: https://pubmed.ncbi.nlm.nih.gov/25750761/

366. Wysham C, Lush C, Zhang B, Maier H, Wilhelm K. Effect of pramlintide as an adjunct to basal insulin on markers of cardiovascular risk in patients with type 2 diabetes. Current Medical Research and Opinion [Internet]. 2007;24(1). Available from: https://pubmed.ncbi.nlm.nih.gov/18031595/

367. Arvanitakis Z, Wilson RS, Bienias JL, Evans DA, Bennett DA. Diabetes Mellitus and Risk of Alzheimer Disease and Decline in Cognitive Function. Archives of Neurology [Internet]. 2004 Aug;61(5):661–6. Available from: https://jamanetwork.com/journals/jamaneurology/fullarticle/785863

368. C J, G L, P H, Z L, B Z. The Gut Microbiota and Alzheimer's Disease. Journal of Alzheimer's disease : JAD [Internet]. 2017;58(1):1–15. Available from: https://pubmed.ncbi.nlm.nih.gov/28372330/

369. Cavallucci V, Ferraina C, D'Amelio M. Key Role of Mitochondria in Alzheimer's Disease Synaptic Dysfunction.

370. Du H, Guo L, Yan S, Sosunov AA, McKhann GM, Yan SS. Early deficits in synaptic mitochondria in an Alzheimer's disease mouse model. Proceedings of the National Academy of Sciences [Internet]. 2010 Aug;107(43):18670–5. Available from: https://www.pnas.org/content/107/43/18670

371. Melov S, Adlard PA, Morten K, Johnson F, Golden TR, Hinerfeld D, et al. Mitochondrial oxidative stress causes hyperphosphorylation of tau. PLoS ONE [Internet]. 2007 Aug;2(6):536. Available from: www.plosone.org